Copyright Disclaimer

The information presented is the author's opinion and does not constitute any health or medical advice. The content of this book is for informational and educational purposes only and is not intended to diagnose, treat, cure, or prevent any condition or disease. You should always consult with your physician before altering or changing any part of your medical treatment. Do not stop or change any presciption medications without the guidance and the advice of your physician. Any use of the information in this book is made on the readers good judgment and is the readers sole responsibility. This book is not a substitute for a physician. This book is independently authored and published and no sponsorship or endorsement of this book by, and no affiliation with, any trademarked brands or other products mentioned within is claimed or suggested. All trademarks that appear in ingredient lists and elsewhere in this book belong to their respective owners and are used here for informational purposes only. The author and publisher encourages readers to patronize the quality brands mentioned in this book.

MEET YOUR AUTHOR

Maryam K. Muhammad is the creator and founder of the Heal Thy Life Center, a non-profit foundation dedicated to educating women and children on living healthy lifestyles. As a gifted orator, motivational speaker, and published author, Mrs. Muhammad has addressed audiences of all sizes. Her inspiring words offer practical guidance for women and girls in a variety of contexts and have been known to empower the listener to make changes for the better. Maryam is committed to breaking the cycle of disease in God's women. She has organized and hosted many health awareness events, served on various health community panels as a health advocate ion underserved communities and is currently serving as a community council advisor to the South Side Healthy Community Organization.

Her work has placed her in high demand and taken her all across the country to share her skill set and passion. More importantly, her travels have afforded her multiple opportunities to partner with other organizations, schools, and private circles to touch the lives of women and young people in urban communities that are underserved.

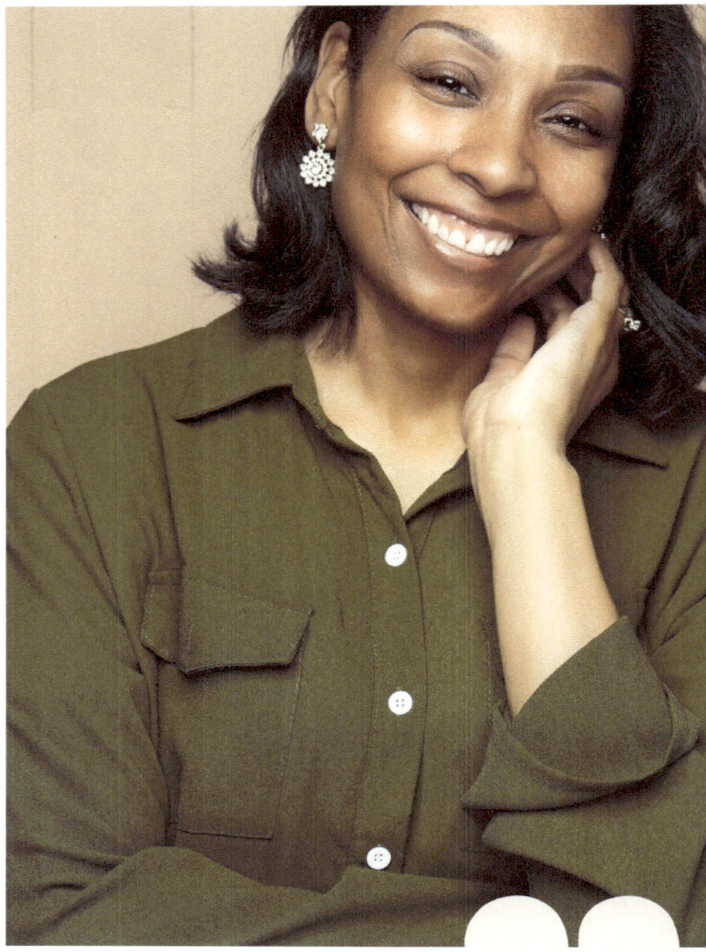

You deserve to live a life free from disease!

Maryam Khalilah

xoxo

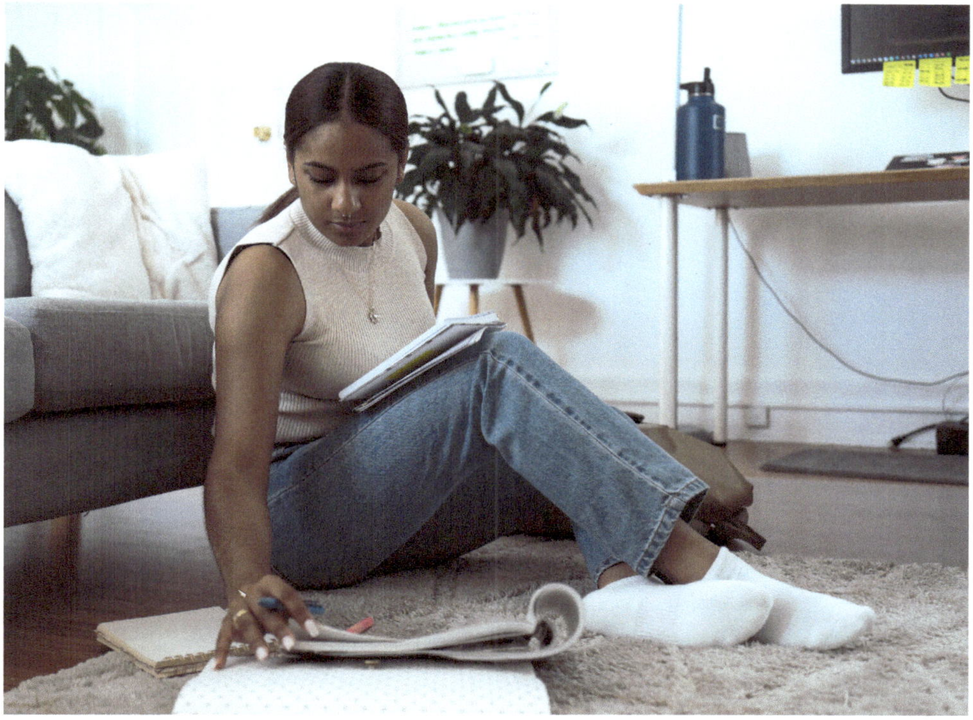

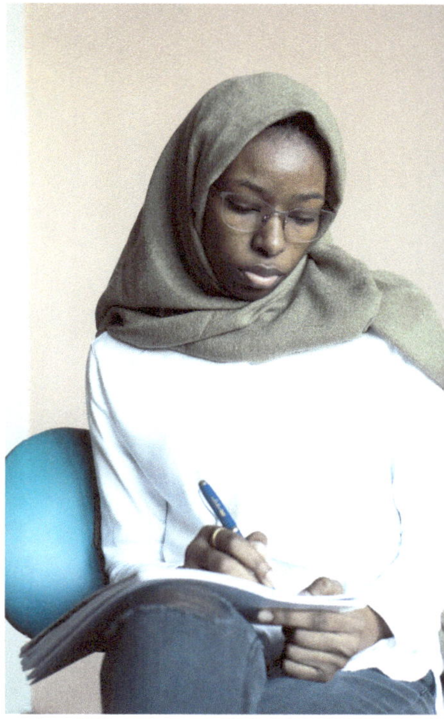

Self Exploration

IT'S ALL ABOUT YOU!

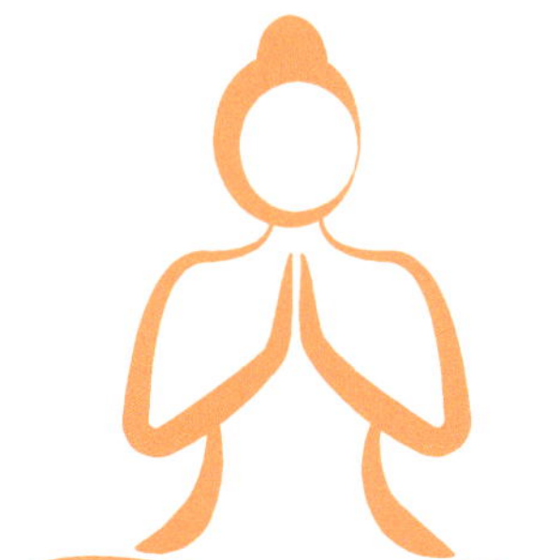

Becoming aware of what's happening in our bodies helps us to make healthier choices. This workbook is all about you! This is your moment to heal your mind, body and soul. Make the choice to stay committed on this journey. Tell yourself constantly that you deserve this and nothing will get in your way! Be honest with yourself. Be courageous enough to accept your weaknesses because when you finish this workbook you're going to come out a stronger, better, healthier YOU! It's now time to strengthen your relationship with yourself! LET'S GO!!!!!

WHAT'S INSIDE

WHAT'S INSIDE

Your Pathway To Becoming A Better You!

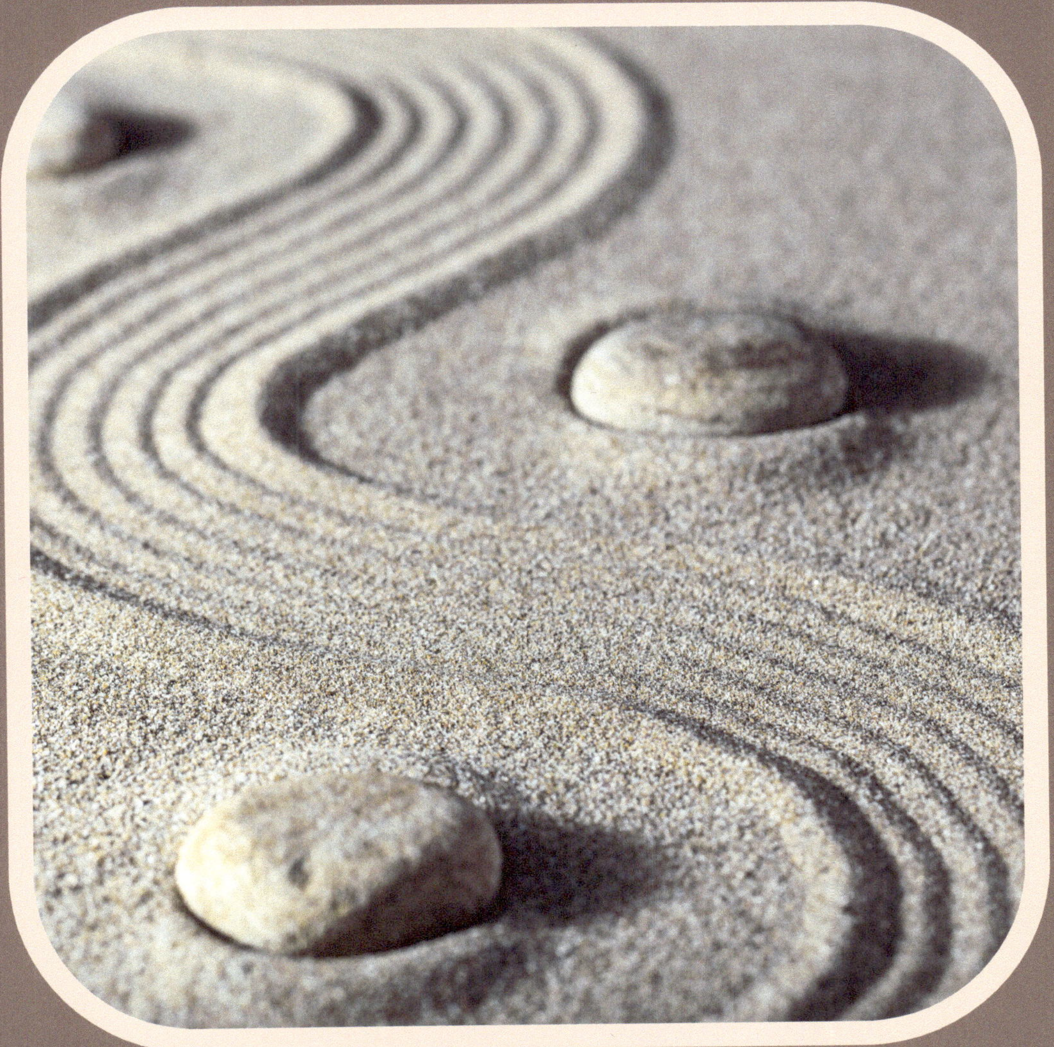

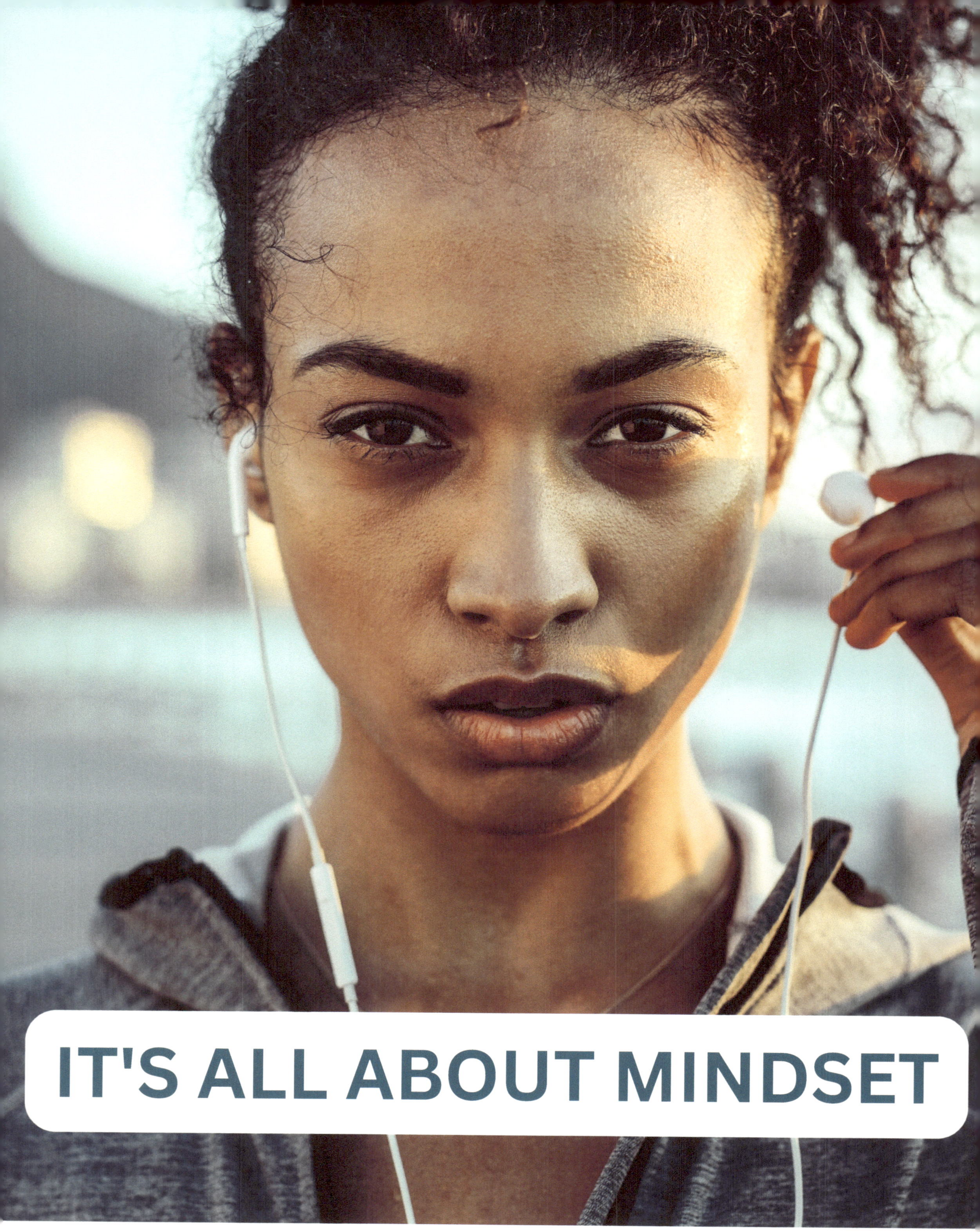
IT'S ALL ABOUT MINDSET

BREAKING THE CYCLE OF DISEASE

The health disparities we face as Black and Brown women are not by chance, it is by design. Our bodies have been experimented on for centuries and now we live a life correcting and preventing disease from existing within us. Studies rarely consider how the historical underpinnings of racism negatively influences the present-day health outcomes of Black and Brown women.

All women get the short end of the stick when it comes to science and medicine. This world of medicine does not invest enough money and time in women's healthcare services. Women lead in the numbers of expressing life threatening diseases like cardiovascular disease, COVID-19, diseases of the reproductive system, cancer and more. It is time for us to invest in ourselves by taking the needed time and attention to improve our own wellbeing. We are capable, we are able, we just need to adapt the mindset that will create a better health future for us all.

Whatever you fear most has no power – it is your fear that has the power. The thing itself cannot touch you. But if you allow your fear to seep into your mind and overtake your thoughts, it will rob you of your life.
– Oprah Winfrey

YOUR PYRAMID

Truth is always found in numbers and you have the power to turn numbers in your favor!

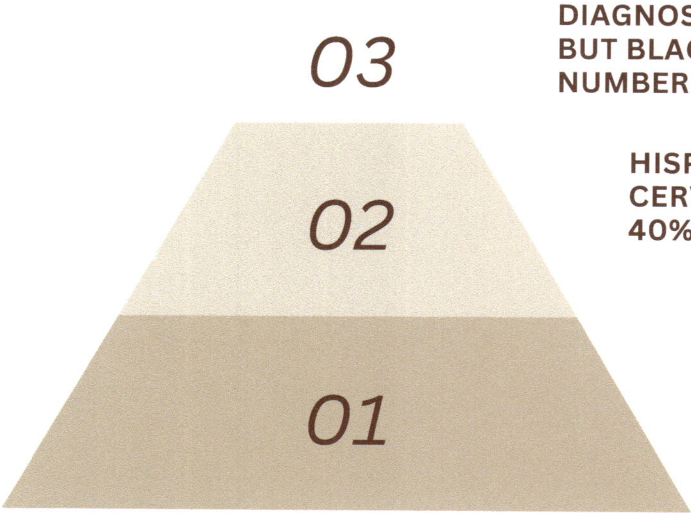

OBESE WOMEN LEAD IN THE DIAGNOSIS OF UTERINE CANCER, BUT BLACK WOMEN LEAD IN THE NUMBER OF DEATHS.

HISPANIC WOMEN LEAD IN CERVICAL CANCER DIAGNOSIS BY 40%.

80% OF AFRICAN AMERICAN WOMEN EXPRESS FIBROIDS BY THE AGE OF 50.

FIBROIDS

According to Mayo Clinic, Uterine fibroids are noncancerous (benign) growths in or around the uterus. Some signs are heavy vaginal bleeding, low back pain, rectual pressure, bladder problems and pelvic discomfort.

CERVICAL CANCER

According to Mayo Clinic, Cervical cancer occurs when cells in the cervix, the lower part of the uterus that connects to the vagina, start to become abnormal. Warning signs include but are not limited to, itchy vagina, unexplained fatigue, lower back or abdominal pain and burning vaginal sensations.

UTERINE CANCER

According to the CDC, when cancer starts in the uterus, it is called uterine cancer. Uterine cancer includes two types of cancer: endometrial cancer (more common) and uterine sarcoma. Some of the signs are abnormal vaginal bleeding or discharge. Feeling full too quickly, difficulty eating, pelvic pressure or pain.

BREAKING THE CYCLE OF DISEASE

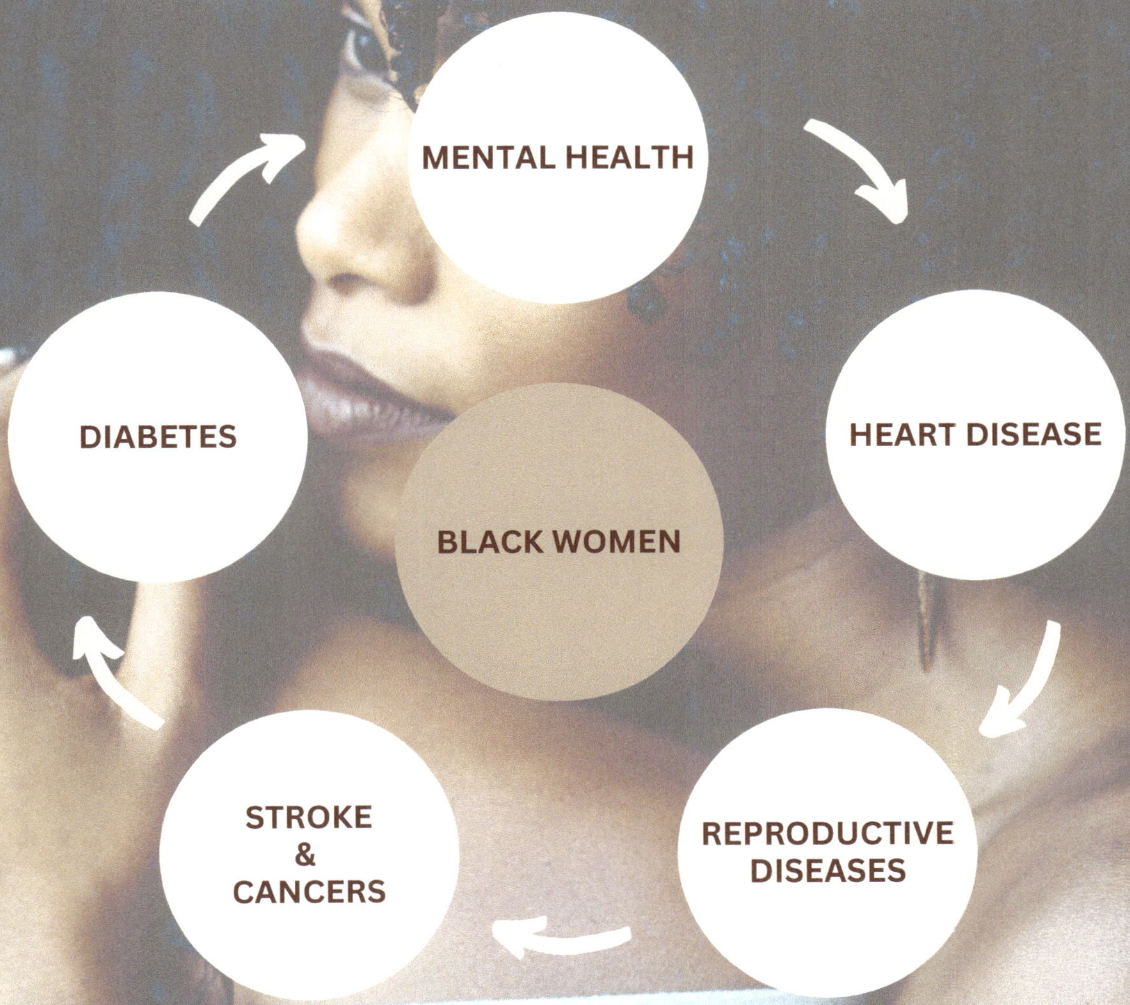

Do you suffer from any of these diseases? If so, write it/them in the notes section. Be honest with yourself. It's time to stop running from being too busy and start to handle the task of fixing ourselves.

NOTES

RECREATING THE CYCLE OF LIFE

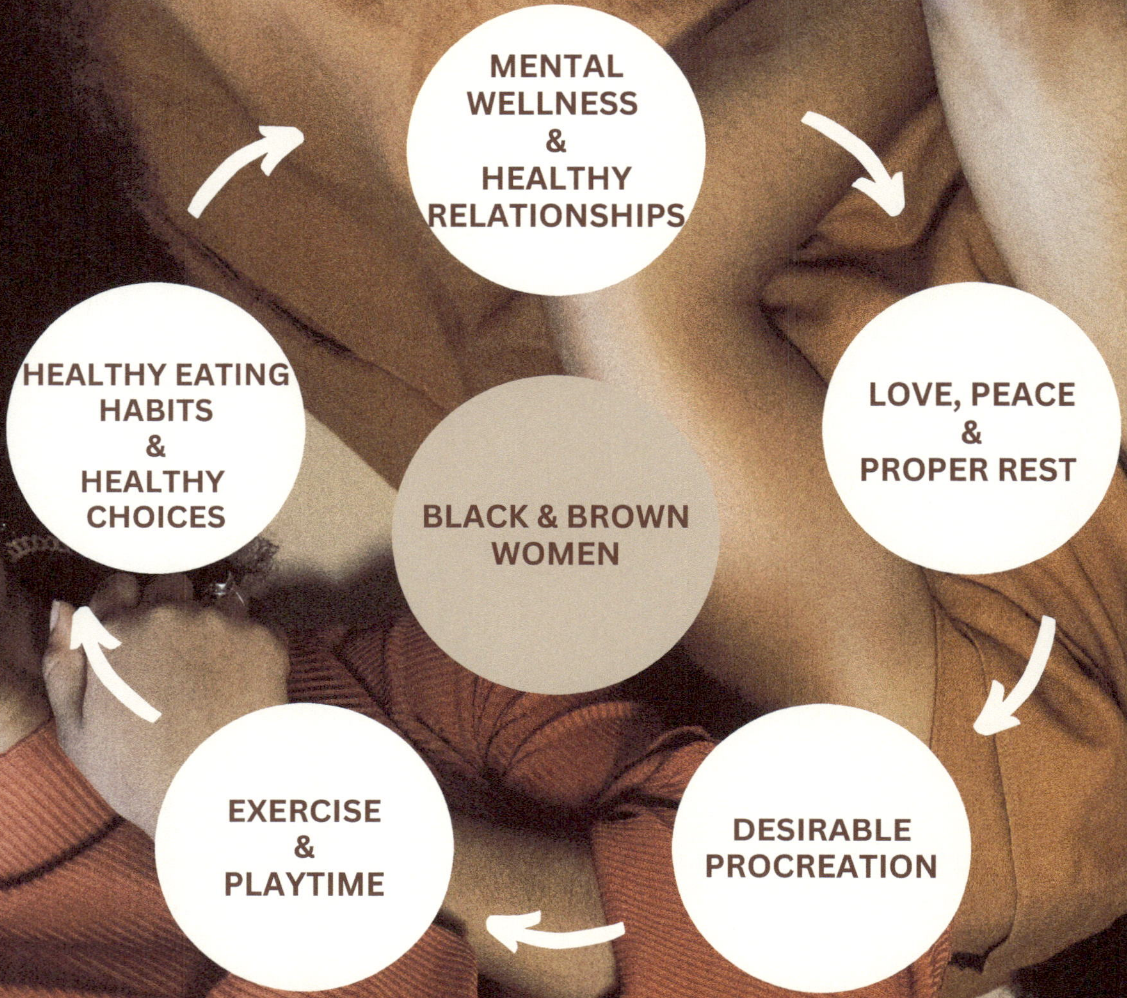

Having a "growth mindset" along with a positive mindset helps us to break the cycle of disease. We have the power to change our reality. All we need is the desire to do so & that will feed our will which will produce movement in the right direction. Being diagnosed with a disease is not the ending of your life. It's a challenge that can be beaten as long as we do not give up the fight!

NOTES

STOP AND BREATHE

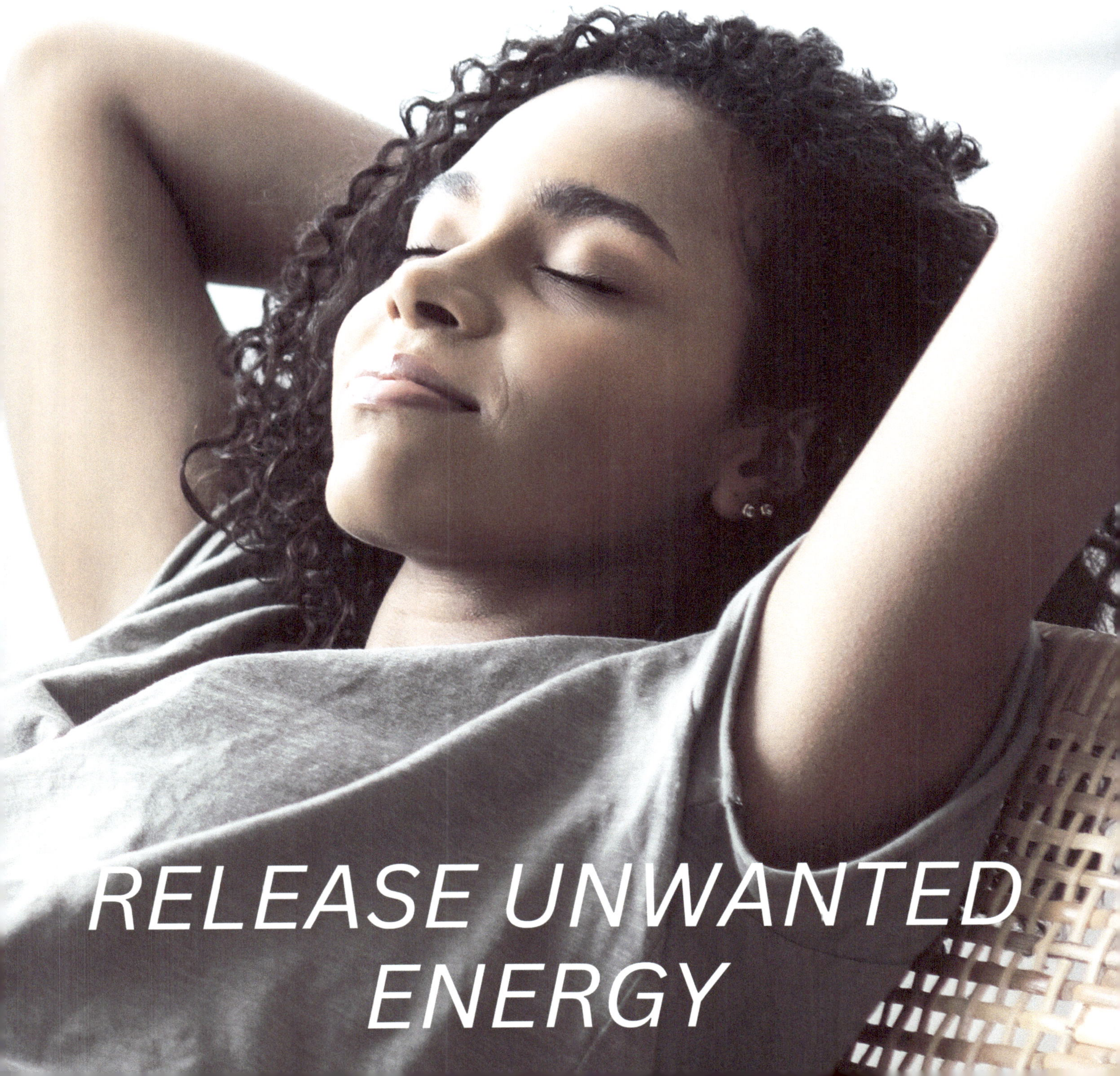

Meditation is a beautiful way to calm and refocus the body & the mind. During meditation, you are turning on your parasympathetic nervous system which is the system that allows us to calm the body down. During this process, your blood pressure comes down, your mind focuses, your breathing slows down and your actions become more intentional instead of being on autopilot.

There are many great benefits of meditation. Some are increasing patience & tolerance, reducing negative emotions, increasing imagination & creativity and most importantly it causes us to shift in our awareness.

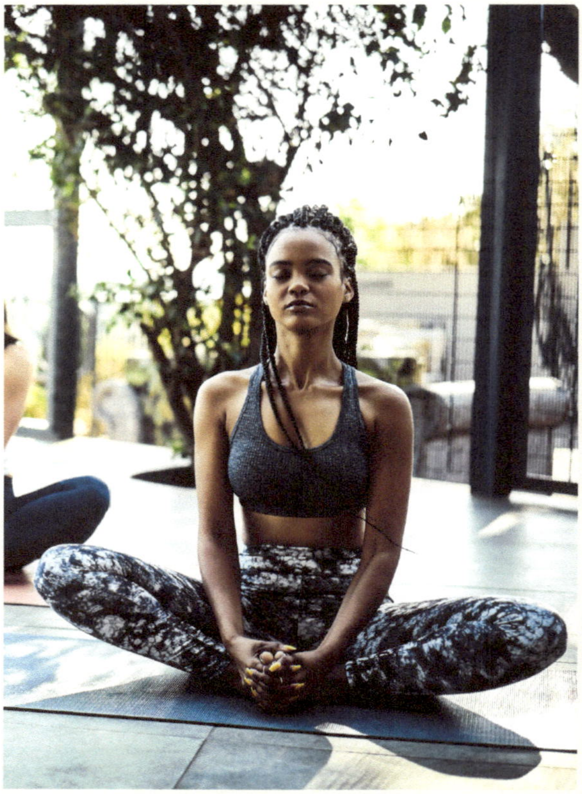

MEDITATION

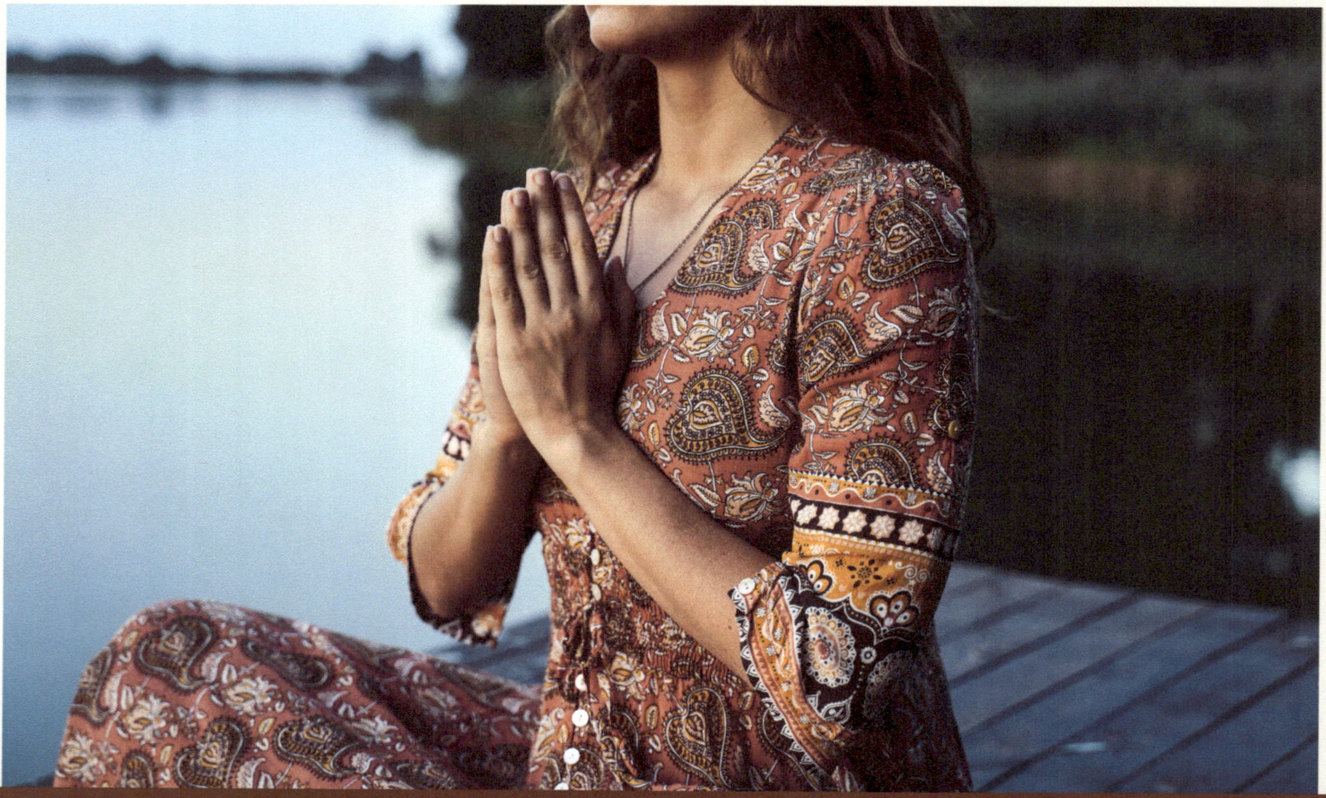

Benefits of Meditation

- Reduced Stress
- Emotional Balance
- Increased Focus
- Reduced Pain
- Reduced Anxiety
- Increased Creativity
- Reduced Depression
- Increased Memory

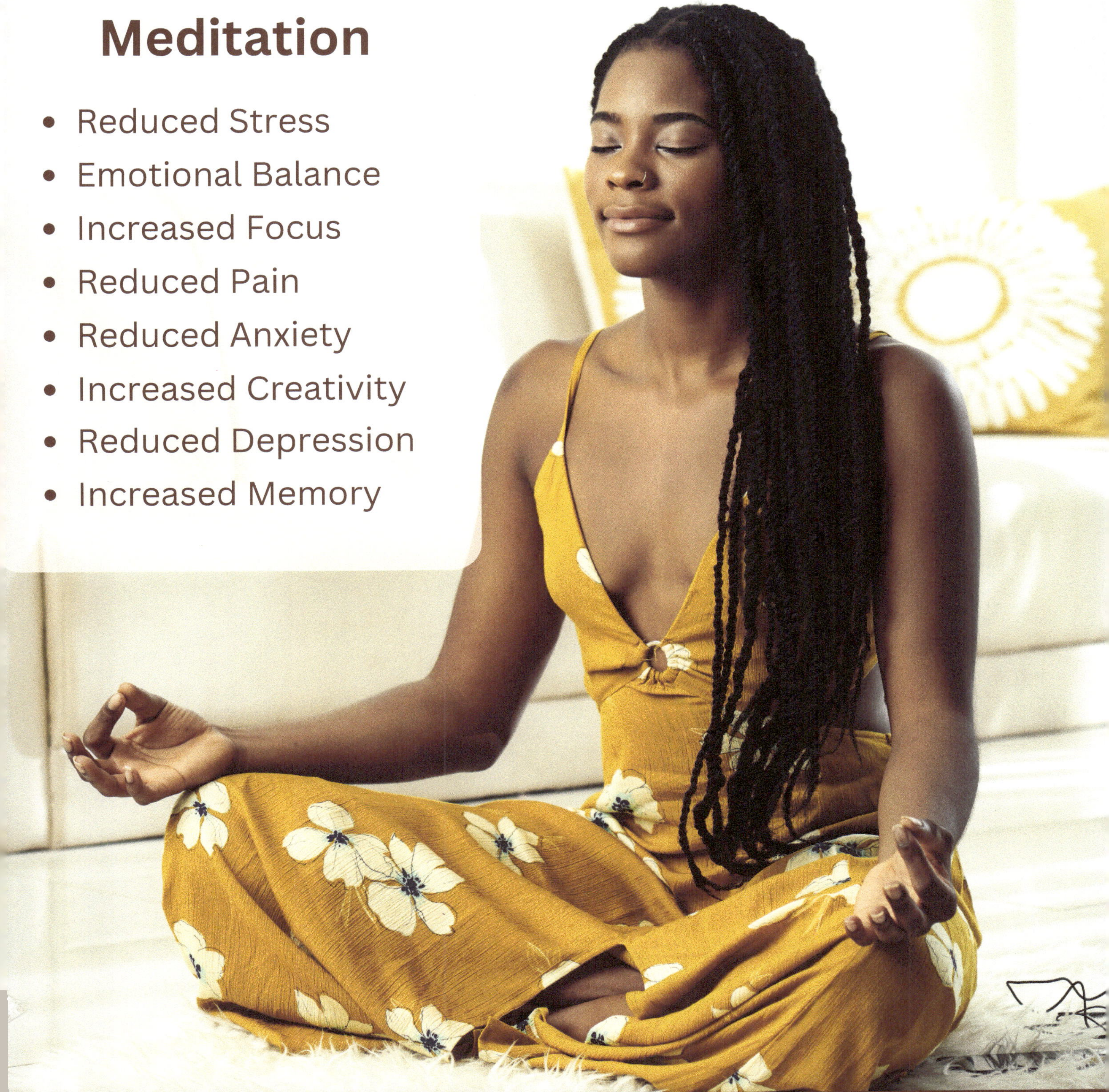

PSYCHOLOGICAL ALTITUDE

LEARN TO LET GO

1 STOP holding on to everything that happens in life. STOP thinking you can handle everything and everything is meant to be handled at that moment. BREATHE and when you exhale, say goodbye to the unwanted, unnecessary, unmerited baggage!

LIVE IN THE MOMENT

2 You can not change the past. Stop living there! It's ok to think about and plan your future. But don't stress out about it. It hasn't happened yet. You still have time to make sure it goes according to God's plan. And don't focus so much on the future, this can lead to robbing yourself of the joy of what's happening right now!

SLEEP WITHOUT THINKING

3 When we fall asleep with the negative thoughts and energy from the day, we put stress on our bodies during the time it should be at rest. When we sleep, the cells of our bodies are regenerating themselves. If you don't allow your body to regenerate itself in peace, you can become a body that breeds disease mentally, spiritually and physically.

BE OPTIMISTIC ABOUT YOUR PROBLEMS

4 Don't be afraid to face your problems. It's important to have a positive mental attitude when you are facing problems in life. See yourself getting through the problem. Visualize your success and prepare yourself not to give up when obstacles come your way.

LOVE YOURSELF

5 Loving on yourself gives you the self-confidence and self-worth we are all in need of. Loving yourself allows you to take care of you. It pushes you to become the real authentic you. Celebrate your uniqueness & celebrate your value. You are a gift to this world. Be free in that which God created you to be. And DO NOT apologize! When you learn it's ok to love yourself, you'll become even more capable to purely love others!

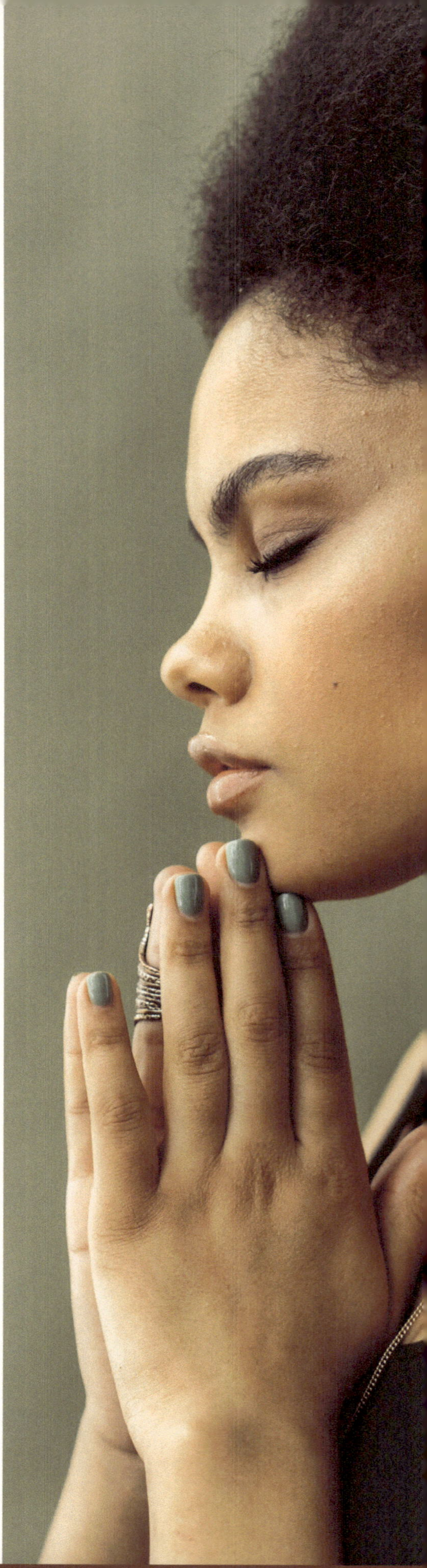

Take Time to Recharge

Taking the time to recharge is all about self-care. Claiming that moment when you refill your cup. This is the time you focus only on yourself and not the needs of others. Don't feel guilty, we all need breaks from our everyday lives. We need and deserve the time it takes to relax and feel better. You are no good to anyone else if you don't take the time needed to recharge yourself.

Learn How to Relax

You'll be surprised of how good it feels to just walk away from a stressful moment and just breathe. You'll feel calmer and lighter. Simple and quick ways to relax can be going for a quick walk, playing some calming music, mindful meditation, journaling, and dancing/singing. Take a moment to see how your body likes to relax and do what is best for you. Just make sure you make time to relax.

Talk to Your Family & Friends

We are social beings by nature. Talking to love ones that you have good relationships with can help you sift through your thoughts and feelings. Sometimes talking out loud helps us to see things clearly and organize our thoughts. Talking to friends and family also solidifies the sense of belonging. Having a conversation with the girls can help us gain a higher since of wellbeing.

NOTES TO SELF

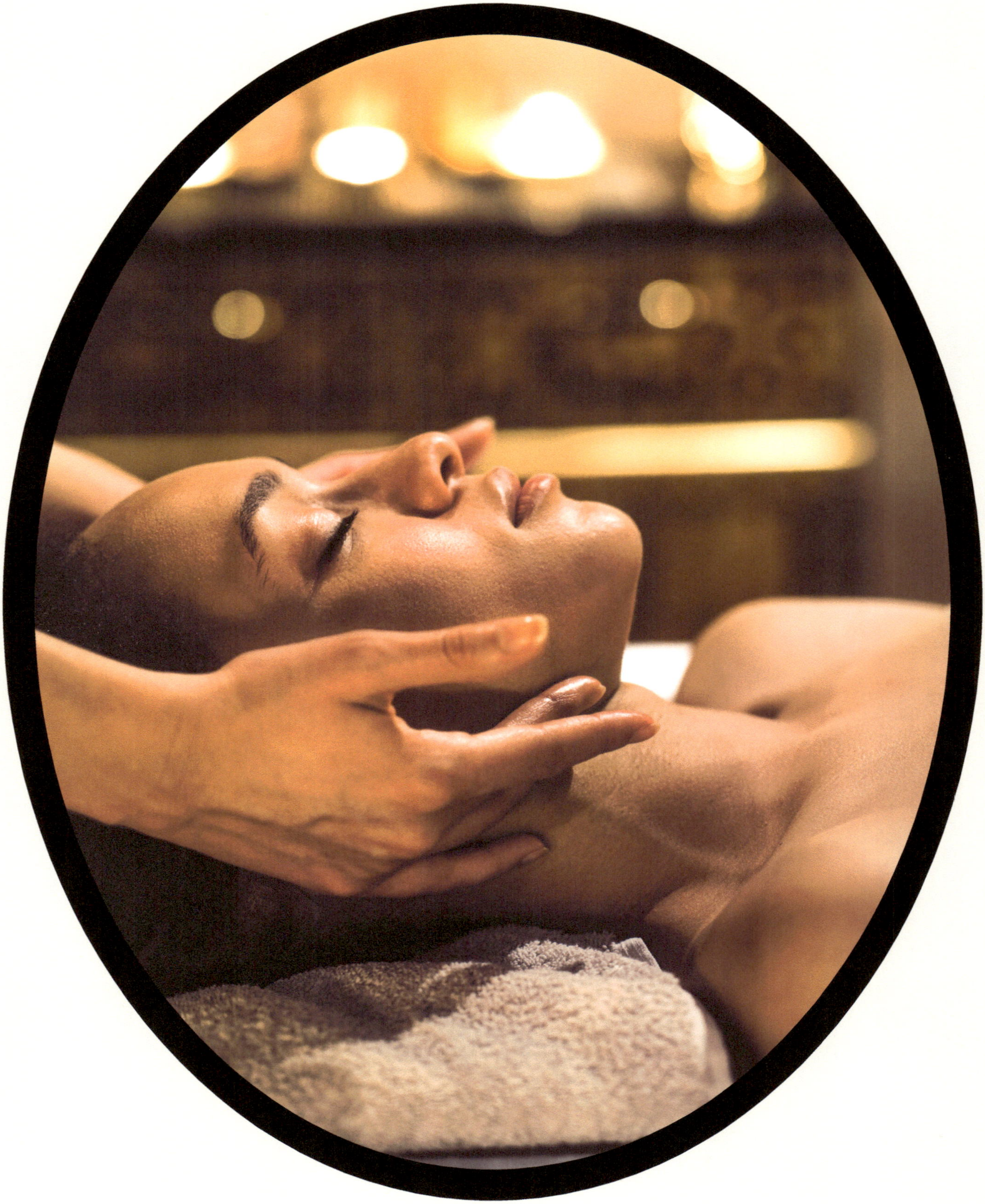

RELAX & RELEASE THE WORLD

Practice Mental Mastery

SELF MANAGEMENT

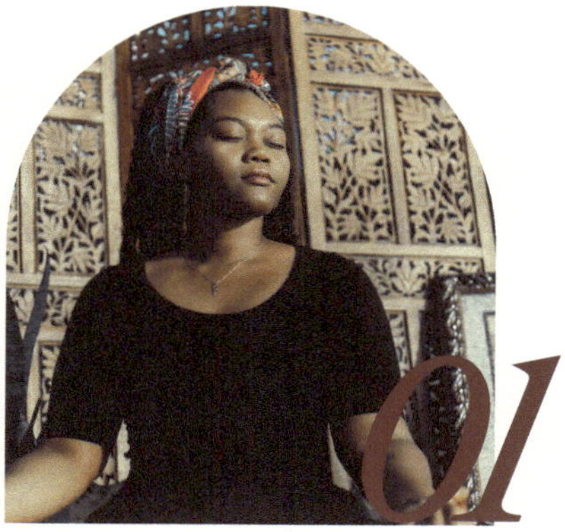

Self Awareness

Our minds often travel between the past, present & future, spending more time in the past. Practice focusing more on the present and what is happening right now. This is your time to focus on you! This is your time to balance your thinking with your internal moral nature. Seek and find who you really are.

Emotional Control

Mastery of self emotions is not an easy task, however it is an achievable one. God has emotions but they do not interfere with His decision-making or how He thinks or acts. We have that ability since we are from Him. Begin to be mindful of your emotions before they reach the surface & control how they manifest. You have that capability.

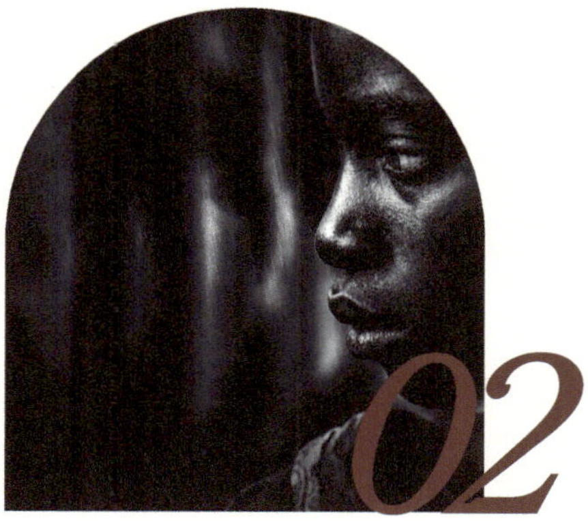

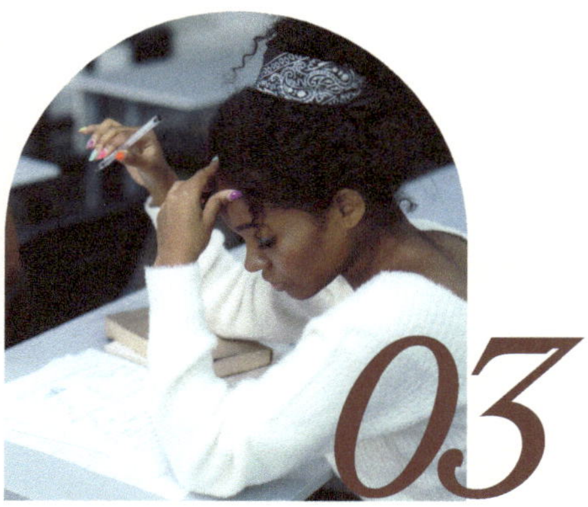

Concentration

When you concentrate, you allow yourself to use the resources of your mind. It promotes awareness & mental strength. When you are focused, you are in full self-control. Silencing unwanted thoughts, improving memory & comprehension. It is extremely difficult in life to accomplish anything without concentration.

Stress Managing

A QUICK REFERENCE GUIDE

Track Your Stressors

When you track your stressors, you gain a better understanding of what your triggers are and how your body is being affected by those stressors. Begin to keep track of your thoughts and feelings. Make note of the information about your environment, the people and actions involved and how you responded.

Develop Healthy Responses

Not all stress is bad. But long-term stress can lead to health problems. Preventing and managing long-term stress can lower your risk for other conditions like heart disease, obesity, high blood pressure, and depression. Examples of healthy responses are taking a moment to breathe, exercise and avoiding substance abuse.

About Anxiety

Anxiety is a normal response to stress. It becomes an issue when it interferes with your ability to function normally. Past experiences like a childhood trauma or a stressful event can trigger episodes of anxiety.

Anxiety has many symptoms. A person can feel nervous or like the world is speeding up or slowing down. Insecurities can trigger anxiety attacks, the feeling that everyone is looking at you when in reality no one is paying close attention to you.

There are different ways to handle anxiety attacks like talking to someone, doing breathing exercises and redirecting your thoughts. Anxiety can be a mind game at times. It is also good to keep a journal of the events. Being mindful of your space and triggers can help you better prevent a future attack from taking place. Staying physically active, making sleep a priority and spending more time reducing stress and stressors is always a plus!

KEY FACTS TO REMEMBER

- According to the Anxiety and Depression Association of America (ADAA), anxiety disorders are the most common mental health conditions.
- According to the CDC, approximately 7% of children between the ages of 3 and 17 years old have diagnosed anxiety.
- According to research at Harvard, anxiety has been indicated in several chronic physical illnesses, including heart disease, chronic respiratory disorders like COPD, gastrointestinal conditions such as IBS, and substance abuse.

Guide for Anxiety

A PRACTICAL JOURNALING GUIDE UNTWISTING PERSONAL ANXIETY

DATE :

____

HOW ANXIOUS AM I FEELING RIGHT NOW?

- [ ] Slightly worried but functioning as usual
- [ ] Madly growing fear and stress
- [ ] Can't focus and overthinking
- [ ] Nearing anxiety attack
- [ ] Losing Control with physical discomfort

WHAT HAS HAPPENED OR IS ABOUT TO HAPPEN THAT IS CAUSING MY ANXIETY?

____

____

WHY DOES THIS SCARE ME? WHAT ARE MY THOUGHTS SAYING?

____

____

Foods That Can Trigger Anxiety

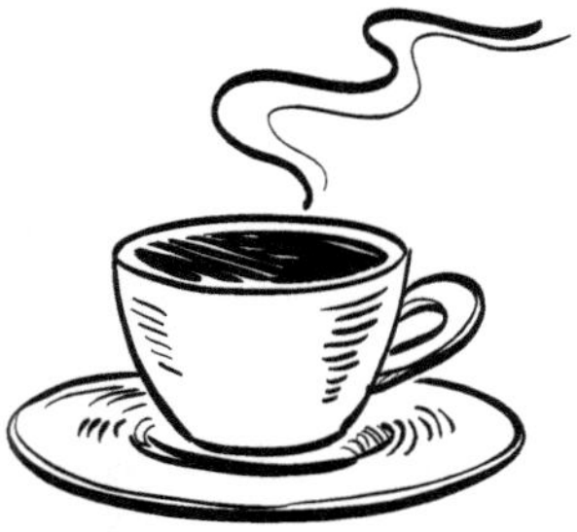

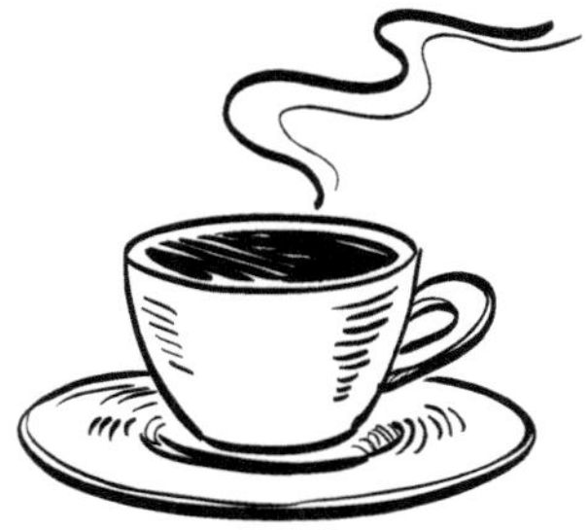

SUGARY DRINKS/CAFFINE | **SUGARY FOODS/TRANS FATS**

Junk food and fried foods, such as pizza, fried chicken, hamburgers, and fries have little nutritional value and are extremely difficult for the body to digest. When the body is unable to digest and process food, excess gas, acid reflux, and other gastrointestinal complaints can produce symptoms that trigger anxiety.

Processed foods, such as canned soups, cured meats, and processed cheeses, contain high amounts of salt. Excess salt intake raises blood pressure and increases the workload of the heart, causing the body to release adrenalin into the bloodstream and leading to anxiety.

Sugar has been linked to depression, mood swings, and symptoms of anxiety. Once the energy boost has peaked, blood sugar levels drop quickly; this leads to lethargy, low mood, and further cravings. The continual boosts and drops in blood sugar levels can trigger the release of adrenalin and cortisol into the blocdstream. This may cause anxiety and sometimes even panic attacks.

Caffeine can be found in a range of products, including coffee, tea, energy drinks, chocolate, and some painkillers. Many people can tolerate small amounts of caffeine, but because caffeine stimulates the central nervous system, excessive intake can lead to heart palpitations, shaking, irritability, and insomnia. In addition, some people are more sensitive than others to the effects of caffeine, so even small amounts can cause headaches, shaking, and anxiety.

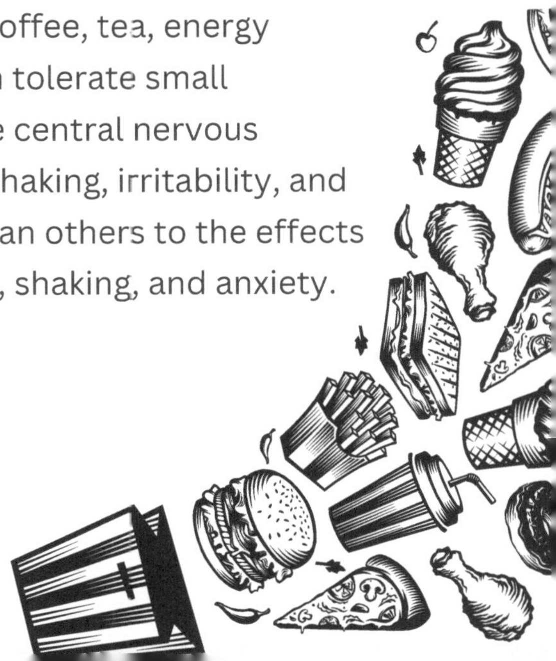

The Intentional Calm Down

SHARE HELPFUL THINGS THAT A PERSON CAN DO TO HELP YOU

TASKS	YES	NO
LISTEN WITHOUT TALKING		
TELL ME THAT EVERYTHING WILL BE OK		
HELP ME FIND WAYS TO RELAX		
TRY TO MAKE ME LAUGH OR SMILE		
TRY TO DISTRACT ME		
HELP ME CONTROL MY BREATHING		
TALK TO ME CALMLY		
HELP ME CHANGE MY THOUGHTS		
STAY CLOSE TO ME		
GIVE ME IDEAS OF COPING SKILLS TO USE		
GIVE ME TIME AND SPACE		
TELL ME HOW YOU WOULD COPE WITH IT		
SAY POSITIVE THINGS ABOUT ME		
HOLD ME OR PUT YOUR ARM AROUND ME		

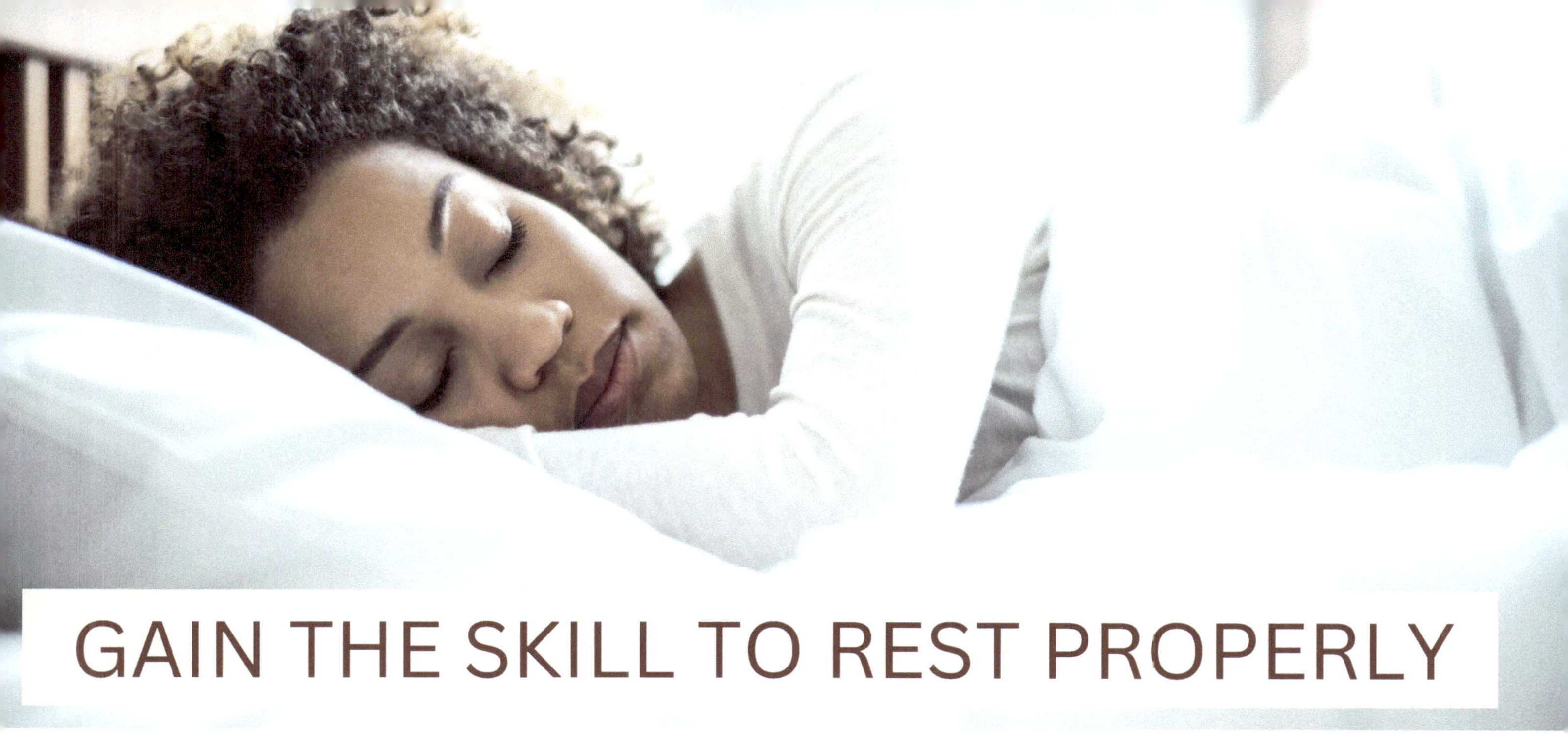

GAIN THE SKILL TO REST PROPERLY

TAKE REST SERIOUSLY

This is a PRIORITY

CREATE BOUNDARIES

Set the time that your day stops and your "you" time begins. No text, no emails, no phone calls, etc. Control how your day winds down.

DEEP PLAY TIME

Engage in mental relaxing habits daily. This can be meditation, painting, swimming, yoga, etc.

DISCONNECT

Decompress your day or the moment. Remove yourself from the current reality and attach yourself to your childhood

READ A GOOD BOOK

Reading lowers the heart rate and relaxes the muscles of the body. It reduces stress. Reading is more effective than taking a walk or drinking tea.

REMEMBER YOU'RE HUMAN

Machines are predictable and boring. You are not. Machines run until they burnout. You are not supposed to. Machines are replaceable, you are not.

! ***No one deserves this more than you do!***

Gratitude Journal

Take A Moment To Be Grateful

SOMETHING GOOD ABOUT YOUR HEALTH

WHAT AM I TAKING FOR GRANTED THAT I CAN BE THANKFUL FOR?

SOMETHING YOU APPRECIATE ABOUT YOURSELF

NOTE TO SELF

Self Love Planner Month:

Monthly Self-Care Goals

1 2 3 4 5 6 7 8 9 10 11 12

Goals:

Why?	How?	When?	Where?

Goals:

Why?	How?	When?	Where?

Goals:

Why?	How?	When?	Where?

MAKING HEALTHY CHOICES IS A PART OF LIFE'S PATH

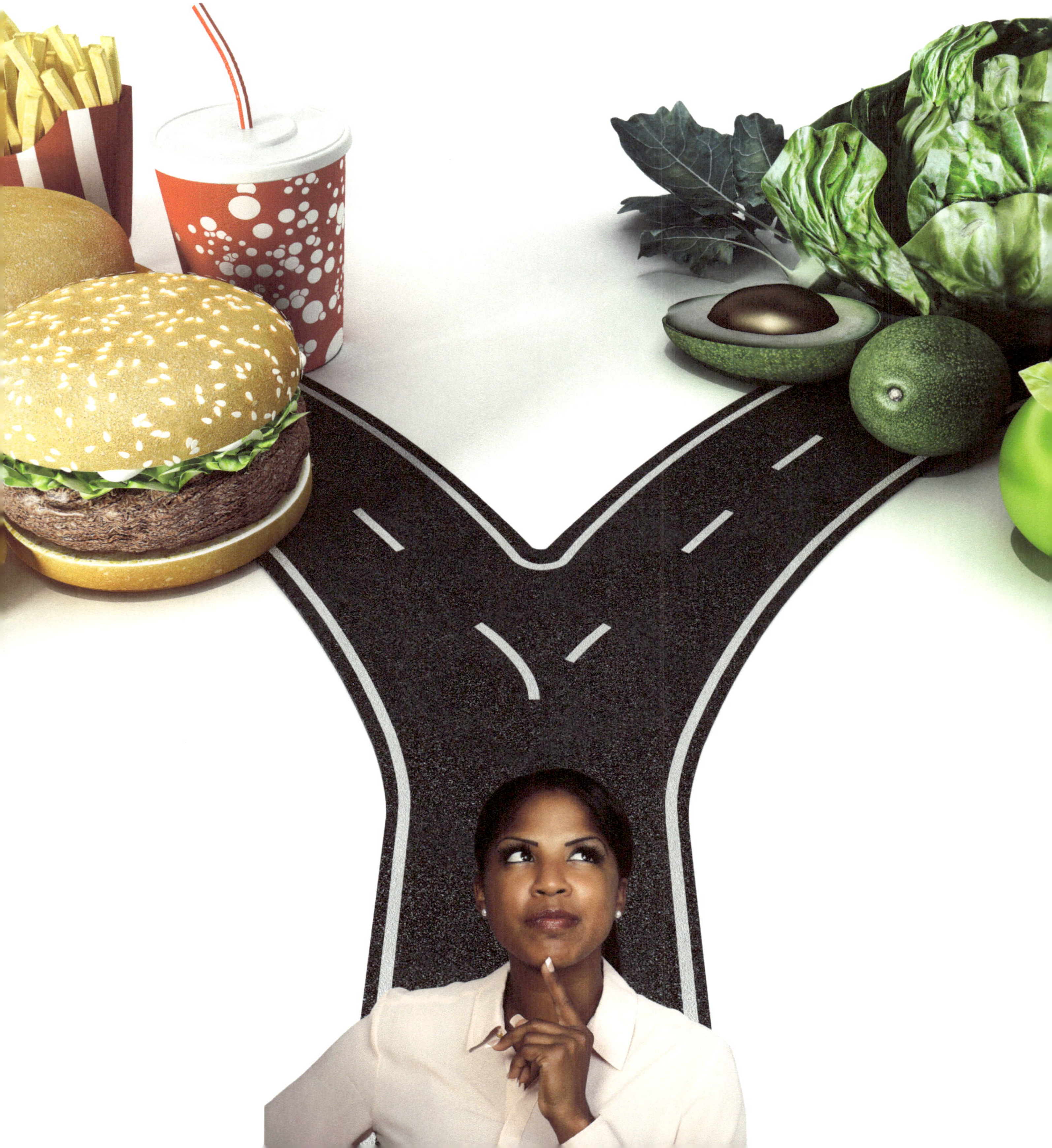

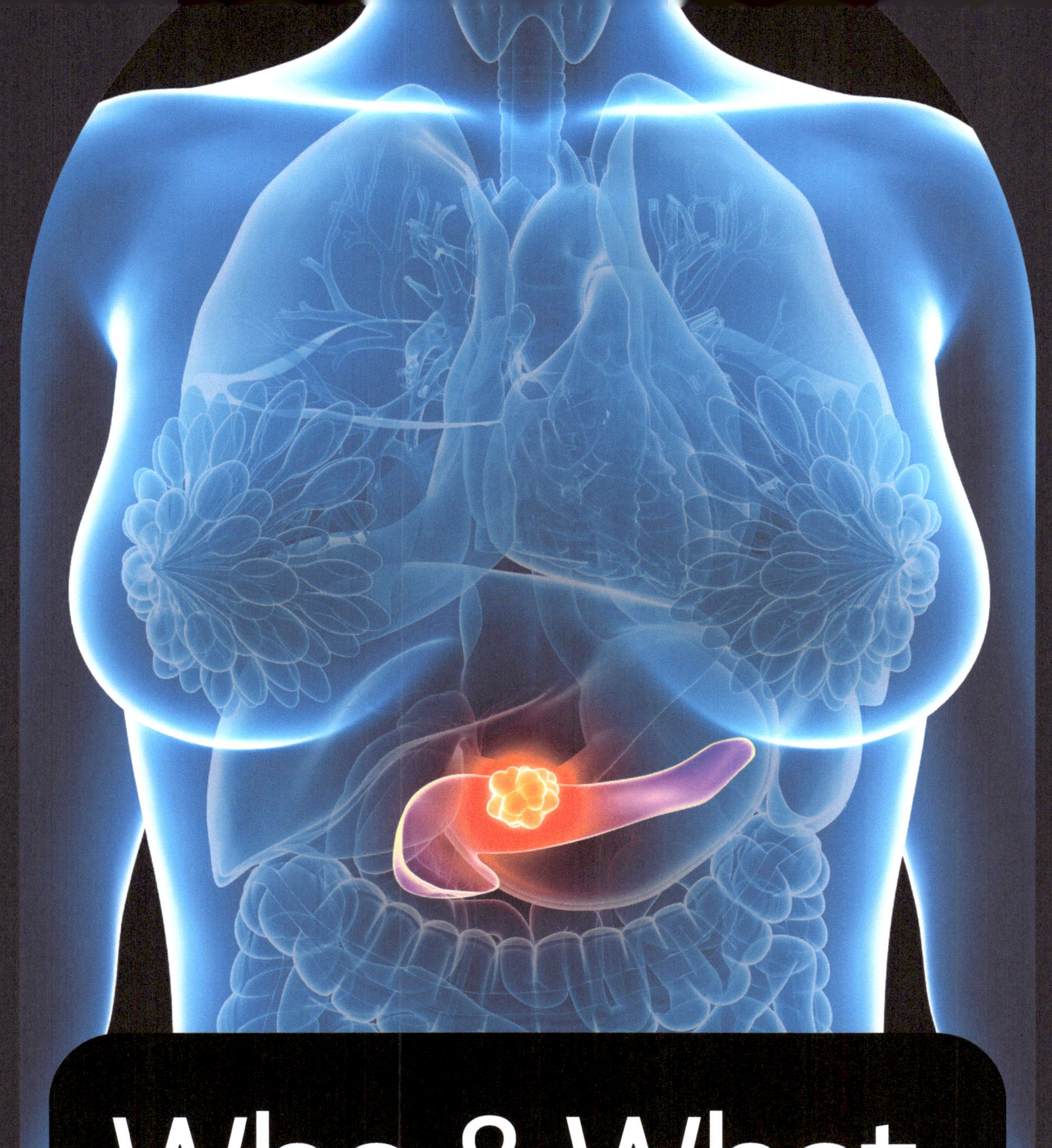

Who & What Is Working Your Pancreas

FACTS ABOUT SUGAR

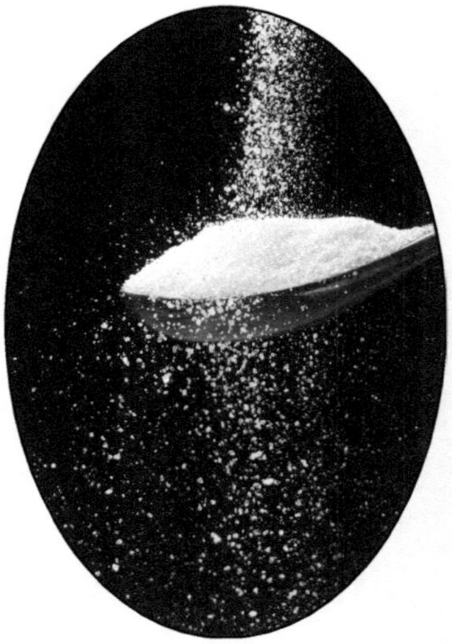

You may already know that sugar can be an enemy to the body. But for some reason, you may not be strong enough to properly balance sugar in your diet. It's ok! You are not alone. Let's work on getting you where you need to be with sugar intake. Read these facts about sugar.

Too much sugar causes the pancreas to produce excessive amounts of insulin. When this happens, the walls of our arteries become inflamed causing them to thicken and become stiff which puts stress on the heart over time.

Foods and beverages that raise blood sugar levels block the production of stem cells that help us to repair our organs, it kills bone progenitor cells and cardiac (heart) stem cells to name a few. We need our stem cells as we age. This helps us maintain a higher quality of living and possibly live longer.

✦ QUICK TIP ✦

Always have fruit, water or tea closer to your reach than candy & soda!

MORE FACTS ABOUT SUGAR

Serotonin is a nerotransmitter our bodies produce to help regulate body temperature, behavior and attention. Sugar interferes with the production of serotonin which has been proven to lead to depression. Serotonin also plays a role in our digestive process, breathing and blood flow. Serotonin plays a crucial role with sleep and wakefulness. It is the precursor to produce melatonin to put us to sleep and it's the key to waking us up in the morning.

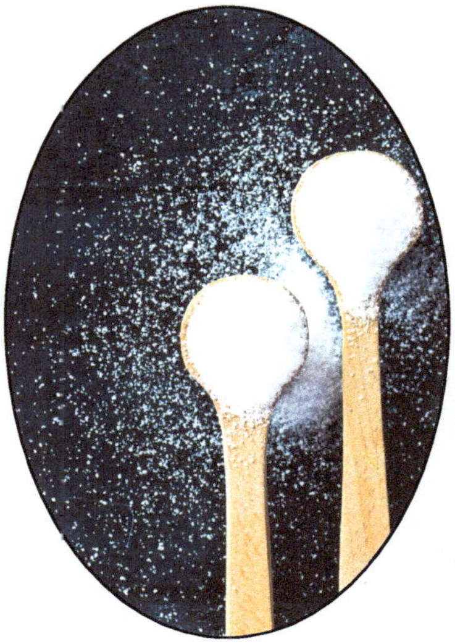

Above average amounts of sugar in our blood stream can lead to fertility issues and the ovaries producing too much testosterone which causes hair loss. It has also been found to feed the growth of fibroid tumors, increase menstrual cramps and create a heavy menstrual flow. Additionally, sugar can cause an imbalance in hormone production and secretion.

✦ QUICK TIP ✦

Add more protein and fiber into your diet!
This helps curve the cravings for sugar!

Eat more natural sugar from your fruits and vegetables. You deserve to live a healthier lifestyle. You can do it! Look at yourself in the mirror every morning and say, "I'm going to make healthier choices because I LOVE ME!"

WHAT ARE REFINED SUGARS DOING TO YOUR BODY

EXCESS SUGAR

We all know too much sugar is not good for our bodies even though we still consume too much sugar.

Our main sources of added sugar are things like sugary drinks, donuts, candy, baked goods, and even adding sugar to our food recipes. We may even find added sugars in breads, protein bars, healthy snacks and tomato sauces.

Excess sugar has a negative affect on our bodies. This is why it is so important to learn the names of ingredients on your food labels that translates to sugar added.

INTERESTING FACT

Making small changes to your sugar intake in gradual increments can significantly increase your overall health.

Other areas affected by excess sugar are your heart, pancreas, kidneys, body weight and even your sexual health.

You have the ability to make healthy lifelong changes. Sometimes we just need the knowledge on how and the right motivation that increases our willpower!

1

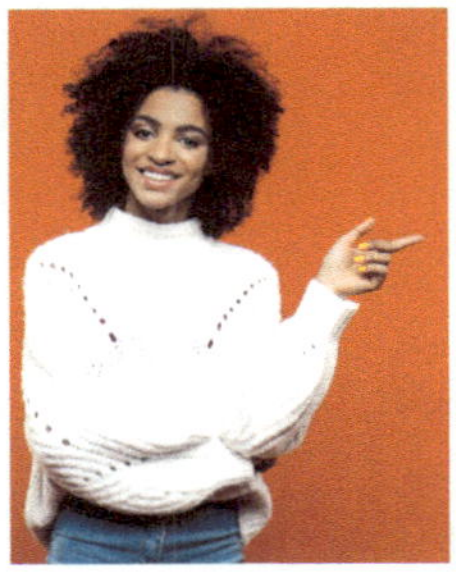

YOUR BRAIN

Sugar gives your brain a temporary "feel good" high that crashes shortly after consumption leading to future cravings. Bring back the balance of the pleasure chemical of the brain with fruits and vegetables.

2

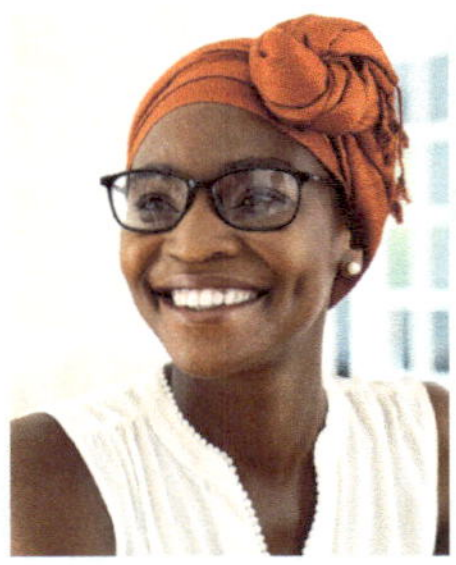

YOUR TEETH

YUP it's true! Sugar rottens the teeth. Bacteria that causes cavities love to feed on sugar hanging out in your mouth.

3

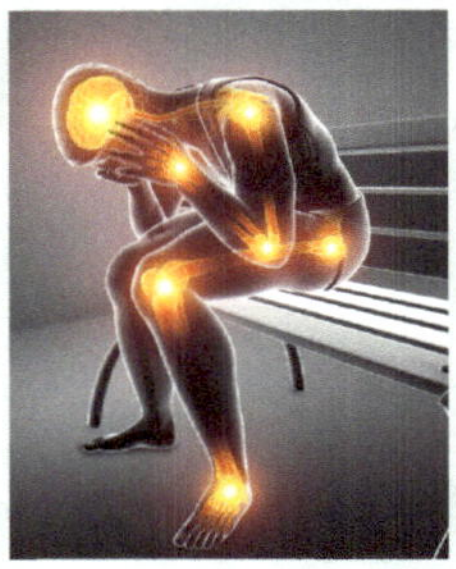

YOUR JOINTS

Eating lots of sugar causes inflammation in the body. This worsens joint pain and increases the chances of developing rheumatoid arthritis.

4

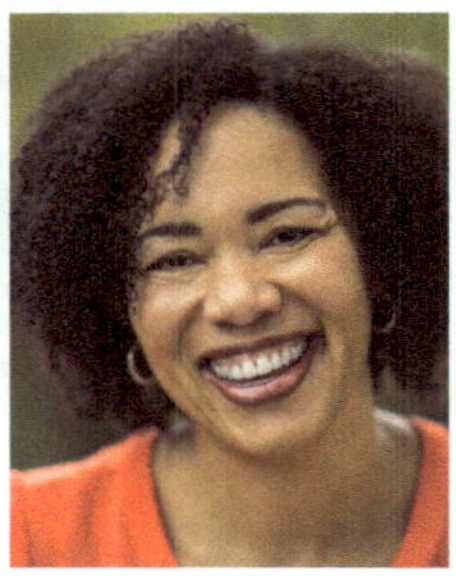

YOUR SKIN

Excess sugar in the body attracts proteins into the blood stream that increases the aging of your skin. These molecules are called AGES. Don't let black crack!

5

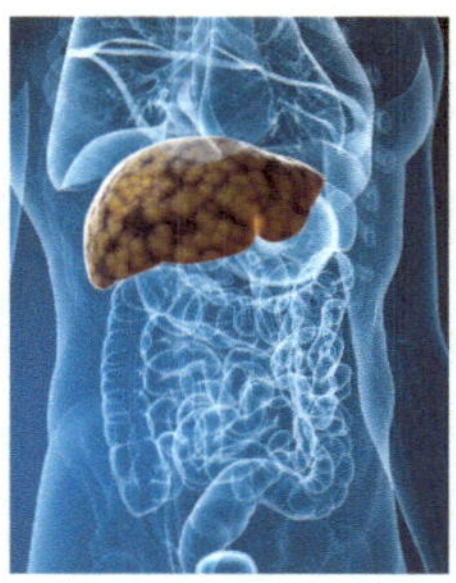

YOUR LIVER

Large amounts of fructose (type of sugar) can damage the liver. The liver transforms excess fructose into fat which causes the condition "fatty liver."

DO I HAVE A SUGAR ADDICTION?

Read each question below and answer as truthfully as possible. Keep a tally of your points and add them up when you're finished.

WHEN DO YOU CRAVE SOMETHING SWEET?

- +1 Every now and then but never daily
- +2 Usually only in the mid-afternoon and evening
- +3 All day long

HOW WOULD YOU DESCRIBE YOUR DAILY ENERGY LEVELS?

- +1 Constant and stable level of energy throughout the day
- +2 Experience mid-afternoon energy crashes
- +3 Lethargic after big meals

HOW DO YOU DESCRIBE YOUR WEIGHT-LOSS SUCCESS?

- +1 Able to lose weight easily and sufficiently when I put my mind to it
- +2 Find it difficult to lose weight no matter what I do
- +3 Gave up trying to lose weight long ago

HOW OFTEN DO YOU EXPERIENCE MINOR TO SEVERE HEADACHES?

- +1 Almost never
- +2 A few times a week
- +3 On a daily basis

DO YOU EXPERIENCE FREQUENT MOOD SWINGS?

- +1 No, my mood is fairly constant
- +2 Yes, I find my moods shift, but nothing crazy
- +3 Absolutely! I just can't help it!

DO YOU FIND YOURSELF CRAVING SWEETS AFTER DINNER OR BEFORE BED?

- +1 Never
- +2 Sometimes
- +3 Always

WHAT IS YOUR RELATIONSHIP WITH AN OPEN PACKAGE OF SWEETS?

- [ ] +1 I can have just one and then put the package away
- [ ] +2 Sometimes I forget there is an open package of sweets in my pantry
- [ ] +3 I can't have just one. If it is open, I tend to finish the entire package.

HOW OFTEN DO YOU CONSUME SUGARY FOODS LIKE COOKIES, ICE CREAM, CANDY, PASTRIES, OR OTHER SWEET TREATS?

- [ ] +1 Just a few times a month (or never)
- [ ] +2 A couple of times a week
- [ ] +3 On a daily basis

HOW OFTEN DO YOU CONSUME ARTIFICIAL SWEETENERS?

- [ ] +1 Just a few times a month (or never)
- [ ] +2 A couple of times a week
- [ ] +3 On a daily basis

HOW OFTEN DO YOU CONSUME SODA OR SWEET TEA?

- [ ] +1 Almost never
- [ ] +2 A couple of times a week
- [ ] +3 On a daily basis

MORE ON THE OTHER SIDE

NOW IT'S TIME TO ADD UP YOUR POINTS.

10-13 POINTS
Congrats! Your current relationship with sugar is in a healthy, balanced place where you feel like you can enjoy it responsibly and mindfully.

14-19 POINTS
Sugar doesn't control you, but you enjoy the occasional treat or indulgence. The idea of eliminating sugar altogether is a tough one, but when you enjoy it on occasion it prevents you from feeling deprived. Keep doing what you're doing.

20+ POINTS
Like many Americans, you consume more sugar than you should and it may, whether consciously or not, control many parts of your life. If you regularly consume sugary, non-nutritious foods like ice cream, baked goods, candy, soda, or fancy coffee drinks, you'll almost immediately notice positive changes when you reduce or eliminate these items. Even certain healthy foods might have hidden sugars, so it's important to read nutrition labels.

You may notice an increase in taste, energy levels becoming more constant, fewer mid-afternoon crashes, and you'll feel good all day long. By avoiding sugar highs and subsequent crashes, you will keep your body more in balance.

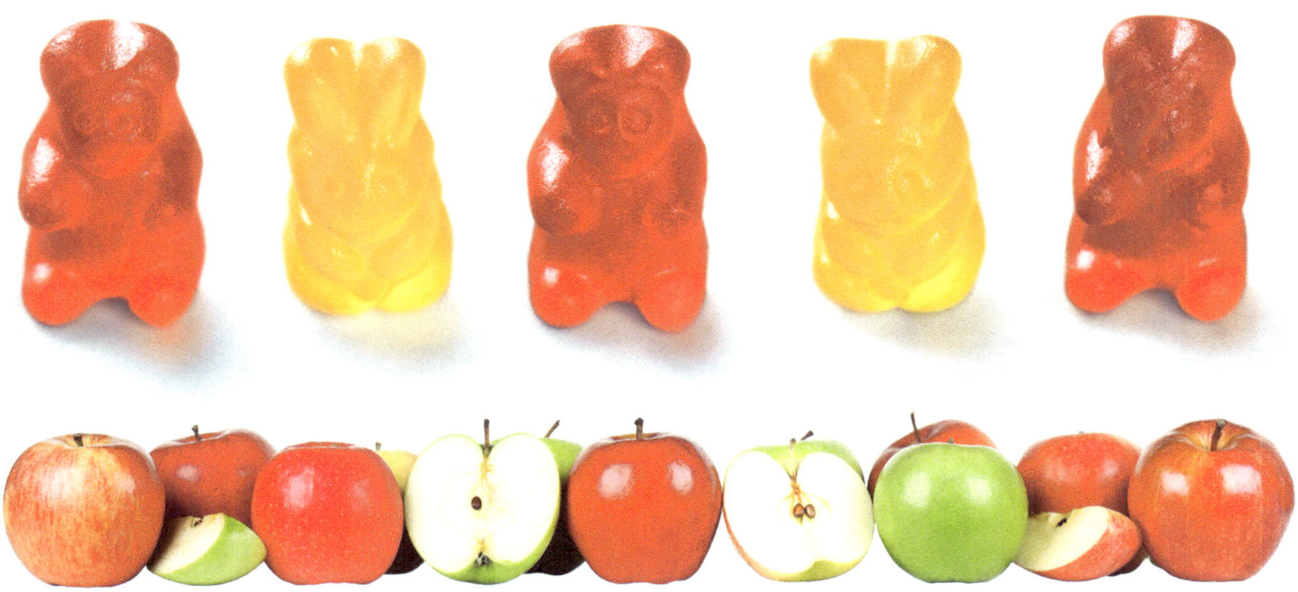

GIVING UP SUGAR FEELS SO BAD...WHY?

- Sugar affects the brain reward system. This system helps us to survive but it is also responsible for addictions.
- Food is a natural reward which can cause you to eat more food, especially sweets.
- Sugar can cause a release of the type of opioids in the brain that causes future cravings.

THE SIDE EFFECTS OF SUGAR

- Per Healthline, the average American consumes 22–30 teaspoons (about 88–120 grams) of sugar each day. The recommended maximum for women is 6 teaspoons.
- Because of the above stated, reducing sugar intake may be accompanied with unpleasant side effects.
- Your body doesn't need added sugar. It turns carbohydrates, fats and proteins into glucose (blood sugar). Natural sugars are fine, which are found in your fruits and vegetables.

Reducing Sugar Intake Has Fixable Side Effects!

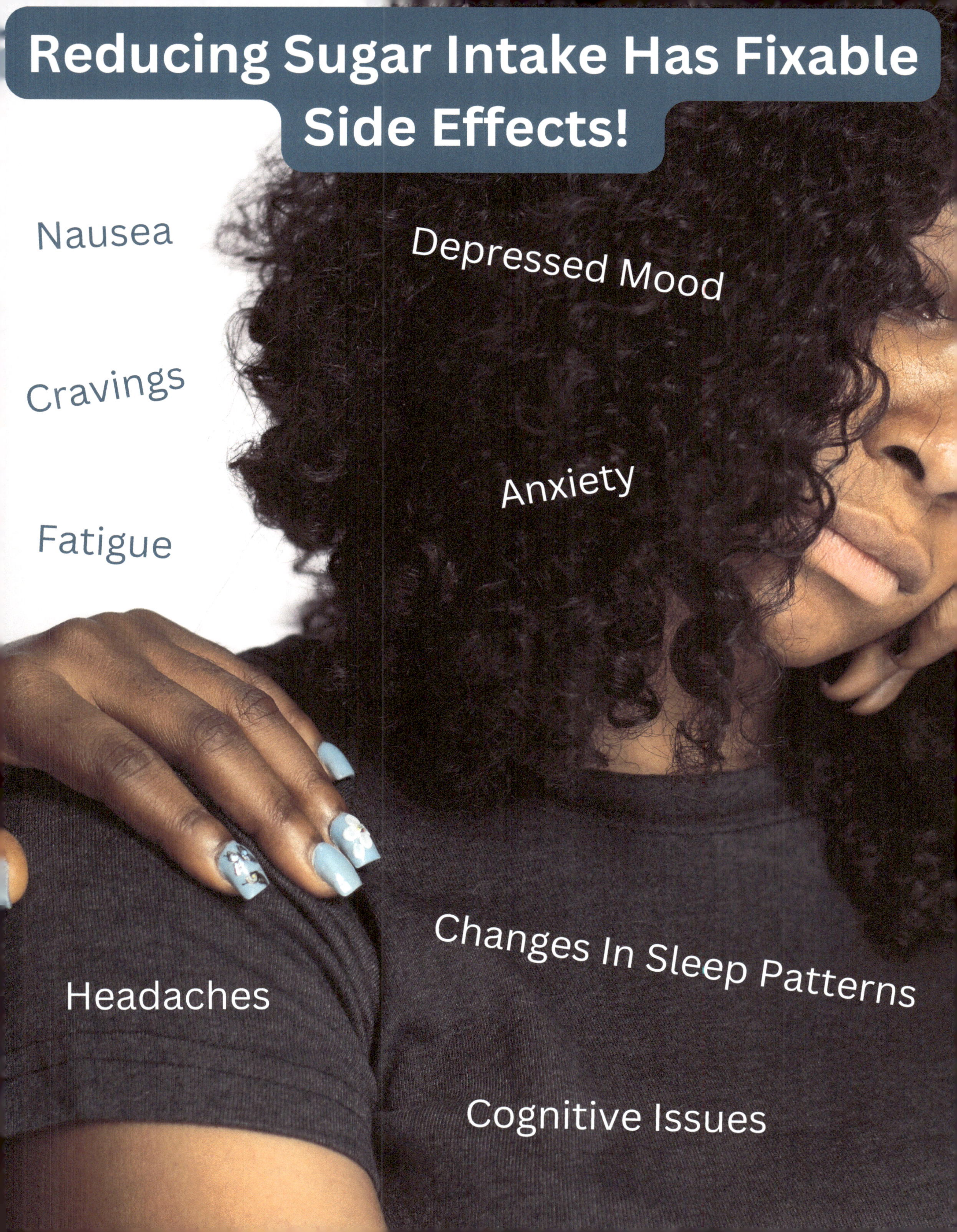
Nausea
Depressed Mood
Cravings
Anxiety
Fatigue
Headaches
Changes In Sleep Patterns
Cognitive Issues

TIPS TO HELP YOU EASE THE SWEETS

Remember...Everyone is different

01 Eat more protein. Protein tends to help curve sugar cravings.

02 Avoid drinking diet drinks. They are not healthy and can raise blood sugar levels.

03 Don't quit sugar all at once. Gradually ease into it. You're more likely to stick with the change and you experience less side effects.

04 Check product labels. Keep in mind, the higher up it appears on the ingredients list, the more there is of it in the product

05 Exercise! Exercise endorphins can replace the need for sugar to hit those 'reward' centers of the brain.

KEEP ADDED SUGARS OFF OF YOUR PLATE

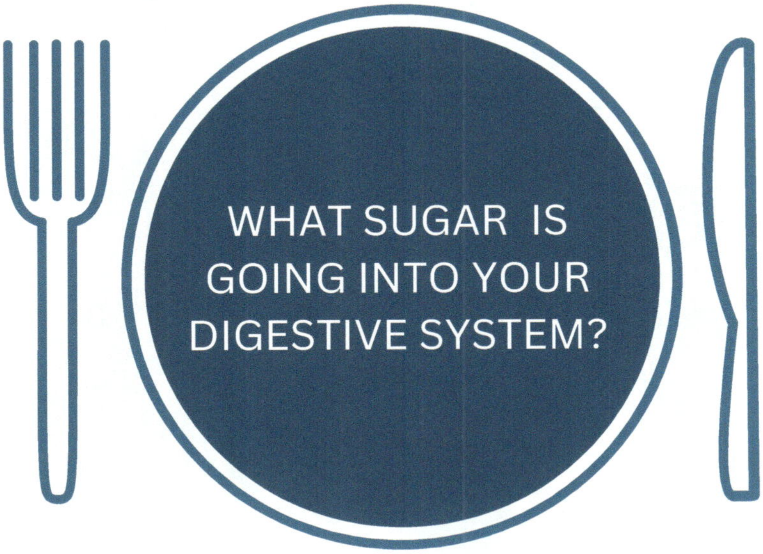

! **Sugar was originally introduced as a spice not a sweetener!**

ALIASES OF SUGAR

AGAVE
DEXTROSE
JUICE CONCENTRATE
HIGH FRUCTOSE CORN SYRUP
ETHYL MALTOL
WORDS ENDING IN "OSE"
ARTIFICIAL FLAVORS
NECTAR
ASPARTAME

FOODS KNOWN TO HAVE SUGAR

CEREAL
FLAVORED YOGURTS
FRUIT BARS & JUICES
SPORTS/ENERGY DRINKS
LOW FAT YOGURT
GRANOLA BARS
FLAVORED COFFEE & TEA
VITAMIN WATER
BOTTLED SMOOTHIES
PASTA SAUCE

HEALTHY ALTERNATIVES

WATER
FRUIT SALADS
GARDEN SALADS
GREEK YOGURT
DARK CHOCOLATE
FOODS HIGH IN PROTEIN
FRESH NATURAL SMOOTHIES
BERRIES
DATES
APRICOTS

YOUR MEAL IDEAS

MEAL 1
- Baked Salmon
- Sauteed Broccoli
- Brown Rice

DRINK 1
Fresh Natural Fruit Smoothie

MEAL 2
- Lamb Chops
- Asparagus
- Brown Rice

DRINK 2
Water/Tea

DIABETES...WHAT'S THE FUSS?

Diabetes is considered to be a metabolic disease which means it's related to your metabolism. It affects how our bodies processes sugar. When we eat sugar, our pancreas produces insulin to transport sugar through the blood.

The exact cause of diabetes has not been discovered yet, but we know stress, eating habits and lack of exercise all plays a major role. The quicker you take the step of declaring to live a healthier lifestyle, the sooner you begin to prevent diseases like this from expressing themselves in your life.

You can beat diabetes. You can beat any disease. It all begins with your mindset. Positive thinking leads to positive actions which lead to positive outcomes. Trust the process and have patience. It may not go exactly the way we desire, but the ending goal is the focus, don't give up the fight!

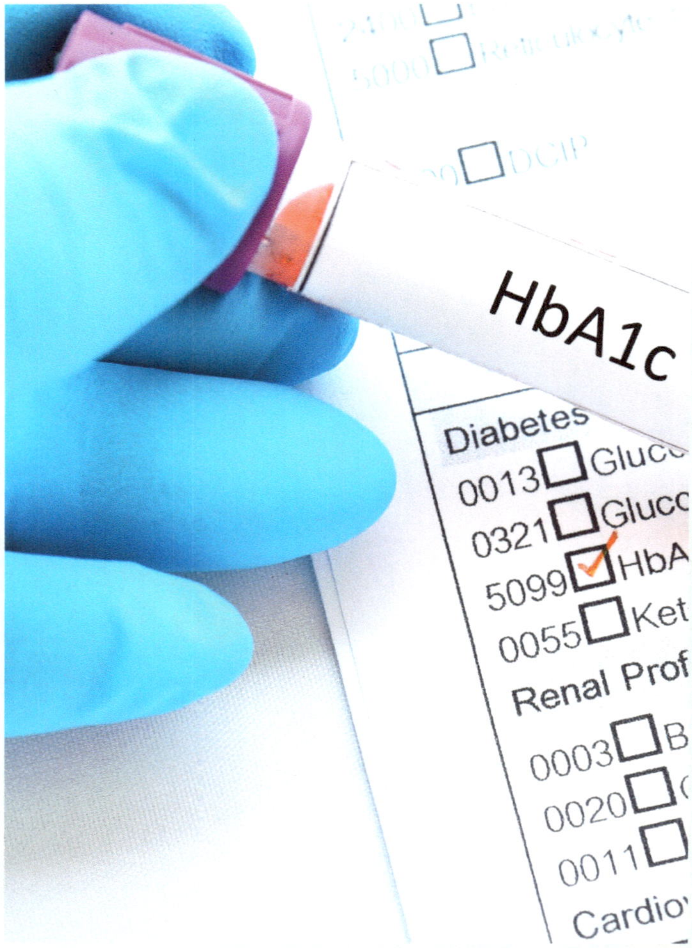

"Women with diabetes have a higher risk of heart disease and other complications compared to men with diabetes"
~FDA.

Facts About Diabetes

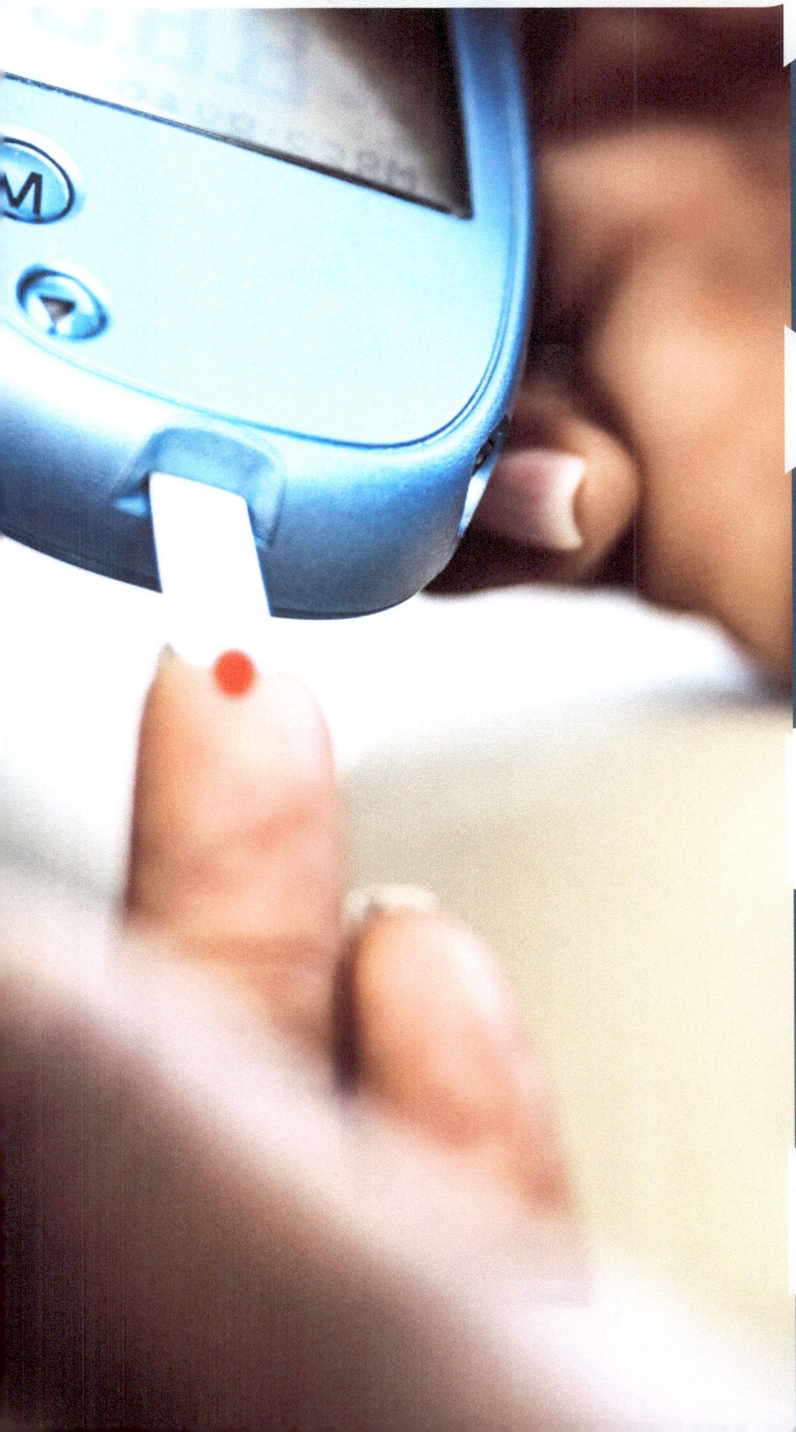

Diabetes is the Leading Cause of Blindness Worldwide.

Adults with Diabetes Are Twice as Likely to Die from Heart Disease or Stroke.

Many Early Symptoms of Diabetes Are Too Mild to Notice.

There's a genetic mutation involved in type 2 diabetes, although researchers haven't been able to pinpoint the exact mutation.

A variant of the so-called Alzheimer's gene, APOE4 is known as type 3 diabetes.

A WEEK'S WORTH OF HEALTHY

DISH IDEAS FOR DIABETICS

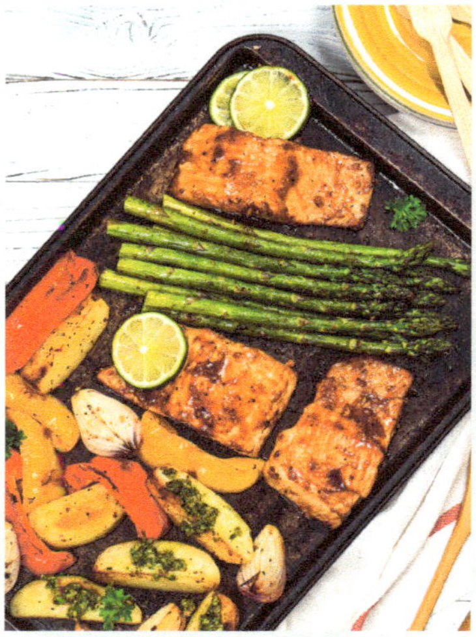

BAKED SALMON

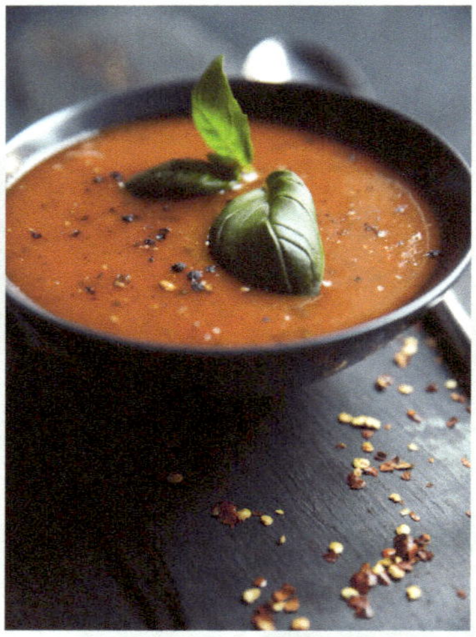

TOMATO BASIL SOUP

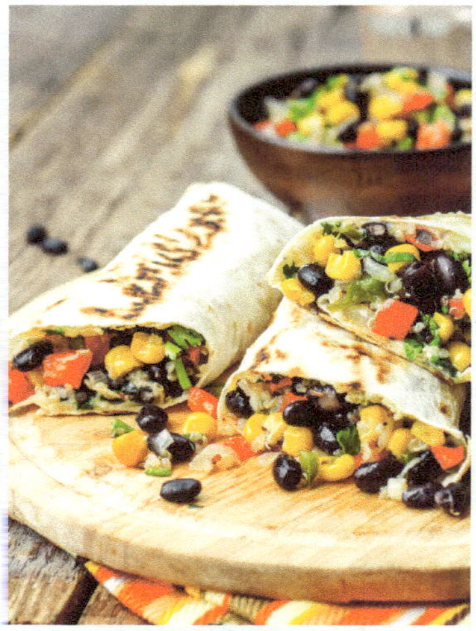

BLACK BEAN BURRITOS

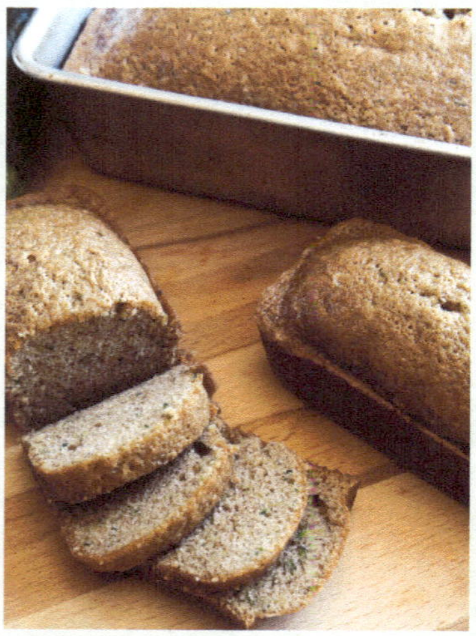

ZUCCHINI BREAD

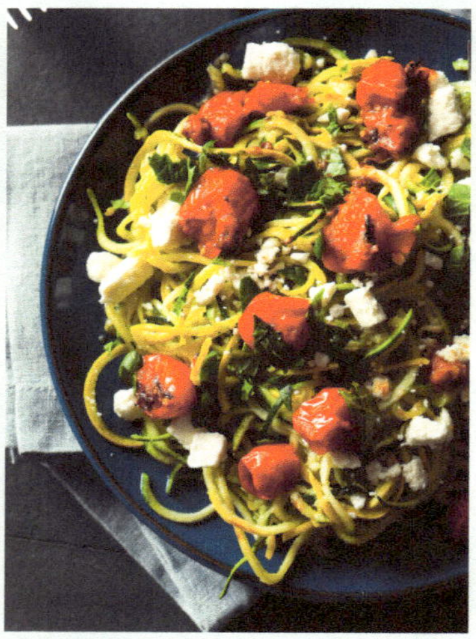

SPAGHETTI SQUASH

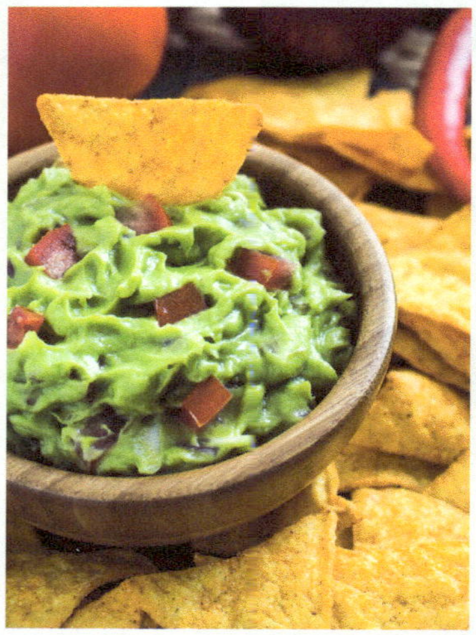

GUACAMOLE

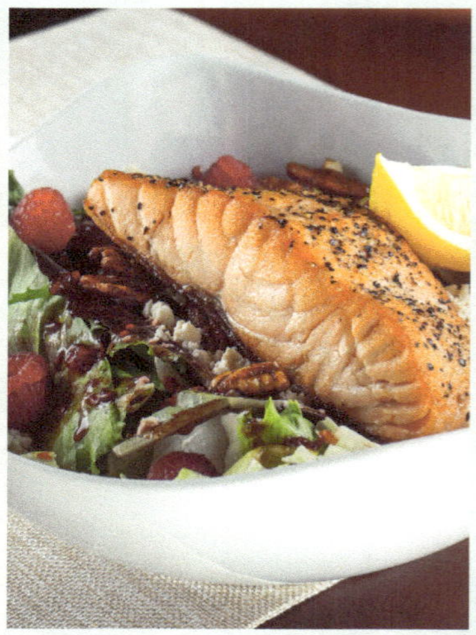

SALMON SALAD

WHAT YOU NEED TO KNOW ABOUT STARCHY VEGETABLES

Starchy vegetables are high in carbohydrates and low in fiber. They are ok to eat, just keep in mind when you have them there is no need to add another starch on your plate and because they are higher in carbs than non starchy vegetables, they can spike your blood sugar levels. Keep them limited to 1/4 of your plate size.

TYPES OF STARCHY VEGETABLES

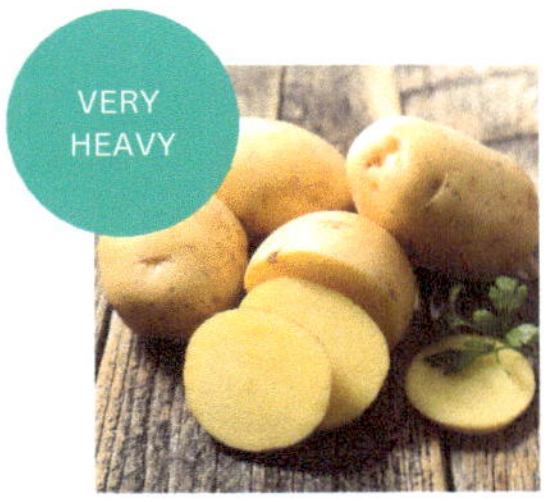

WHITE POTATOES

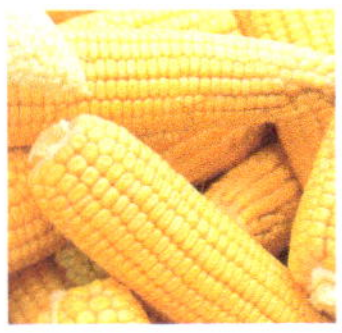

CORN

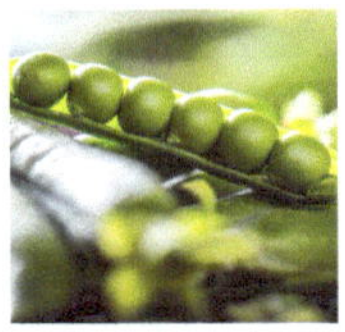

GREEN PEAS

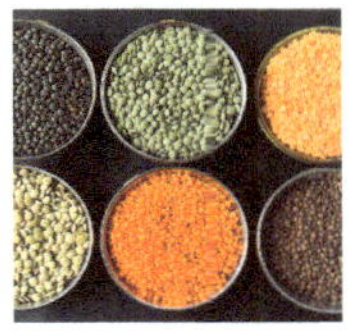

LENTILS

WHAT YOU NEED TO KNOW ABOUT COMPLEX CARBS

1

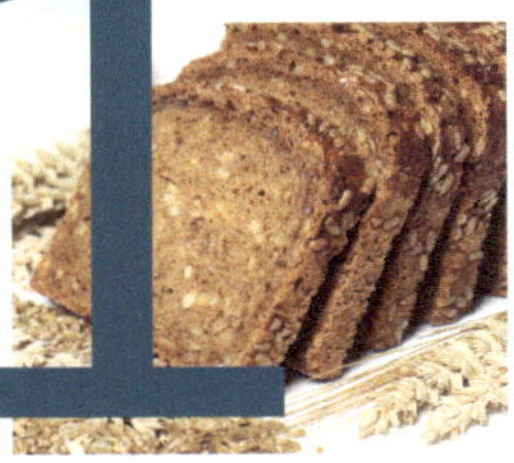

WHOLE WHEAT BREAD

Whole wheat bread is **excellent for your digestive system**. Toasting it makes it more nutrient dense and lowers the glycemic index making it less likely to spike blood sugar.

2

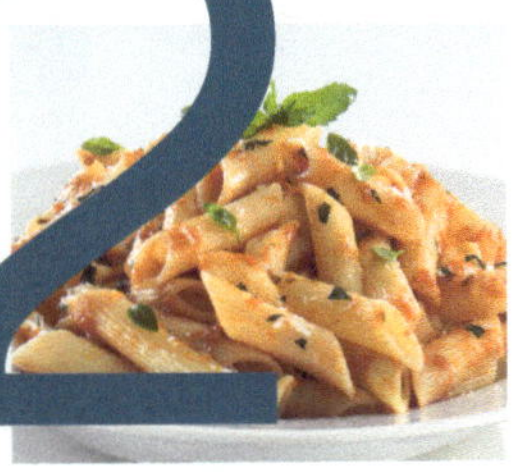

PASTA

Pasta is really high in caborhydrates. This can be a bad thing we eaten in large amounts even if you spread it out over several servings. This may lead to weight gain & digestive issues.

3

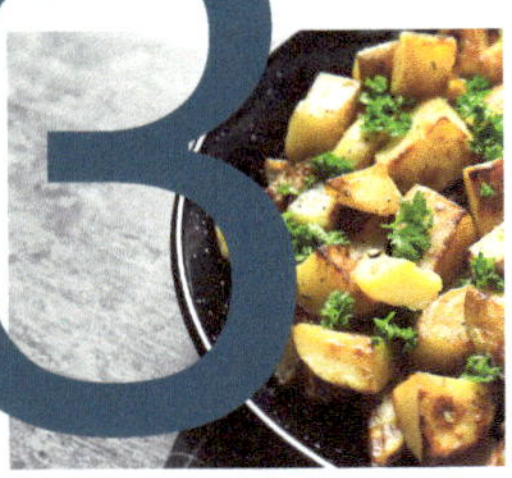

POTATOES

Potatoes are high in the kinds of carbs that spike your sugar levels and your insulin levels. Diabetics should stay away from potatoes. Always remember fries & chips are potatoes.

IMPORTANT INFORMATION

Complex carbs elevate blood sugar levels longer and they produce lasting energy for the body. Complex carbs also promote muscle growth and weight gain and can lead to sugar addictions. Be mindful of your complex carb intake.

EXCLUDE FROM YOUR DIET

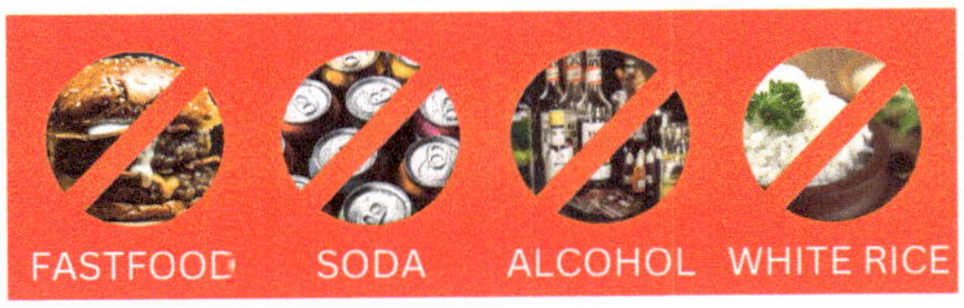

PLAN A PLATE FOR A DIABETIC

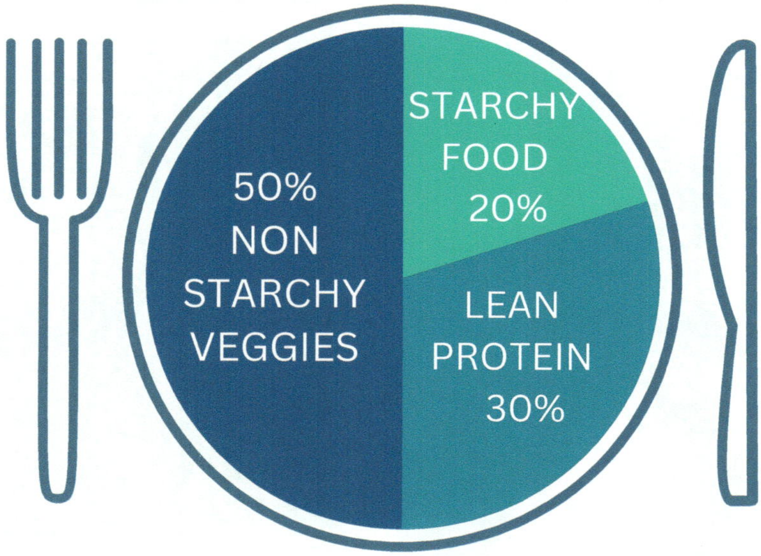

! *Ideas of foods to make your meals with the food portion amounts given on the plate .*

PROTEINS

Navy Beans
Black Beans
Hummus
Lentils
Oatmeal
Egg Whites
Salmon
Cod Fish
Turkey (no skin)
Lamb

NON STARCHY VEGGIES

Asparagus
Artichoke
Beets
Broccoli
Brussel Sprouts
Cabbage
Cauliflower
Onions
Peppers
Squash

STARCHY FOOD

Brown Rice
Plantains
Blueberries
Strawberries
Toasted Whole/
Wheat Bread
Lentils
Beans

TIPS FOR THE DIABETIC WHEN PREPARING MEALS

TIP 1

- Trim fat & skin off of all meats. Buy lean cuts.

TIP 2

- Poach, steam, grill, boil or bake foods rather than cooking with added fat.

TIP 3

- Prepare whole foods & not so much processed foods.

TIP 4

- Stay away from drinks with added sugars like sodas, juice & sports drinks.

MINDFULNESS PRACTICES

Being mindful is being intensely aware of what you are feeling, smelling, hearing, seeing & thinking at the present moment without judgement.

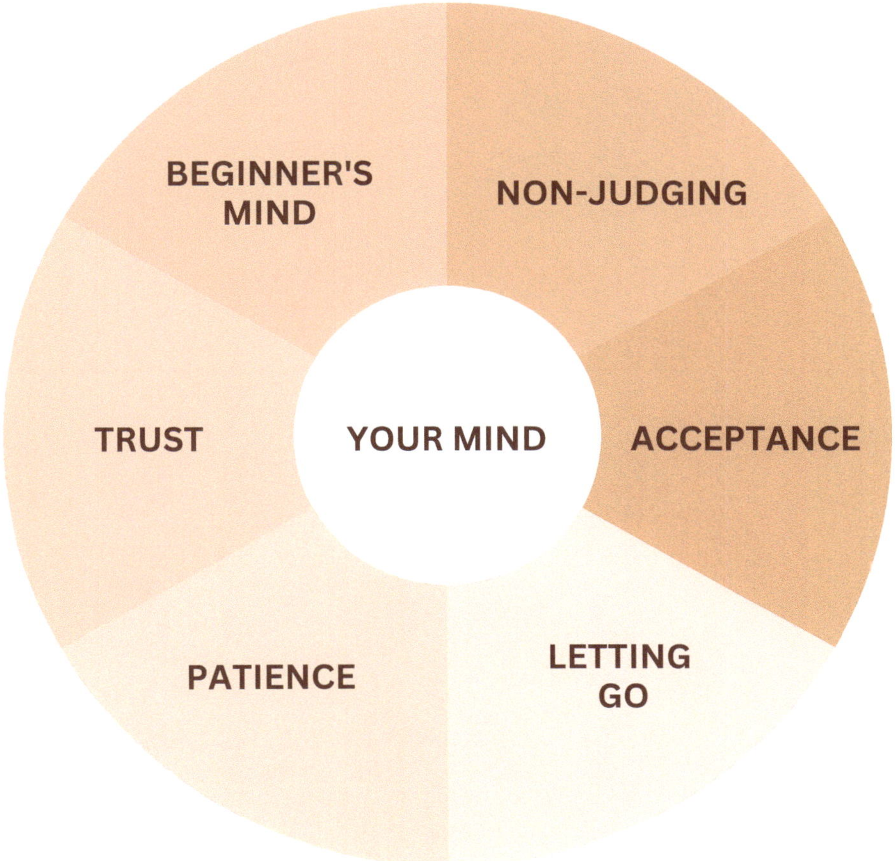

- **Non-judging ~ being an impartial witness to your own experience.**
- **Acceptance ~ Seeing things as they actually are in the moment. Stop denying the factual.**
- **Letting Go- Some things just need to be released from your mind. Every night, when we go to sleep, we let go. So you're already doing it, just become more intentional with this while you are awake.**
- **Patience ~ Let things unravel in their own time.**
- **Trust ~ Create a level of trust in yourself and your feelings.**
- **Beginner's mind ~ Being able to look at things as if it is the first time they occurred. Treat each moment uniquely. See things as they are without past perceptions or the idea that you already know.**

Adapted from Full Catastrophe Living by Jon Kabat-Zinn

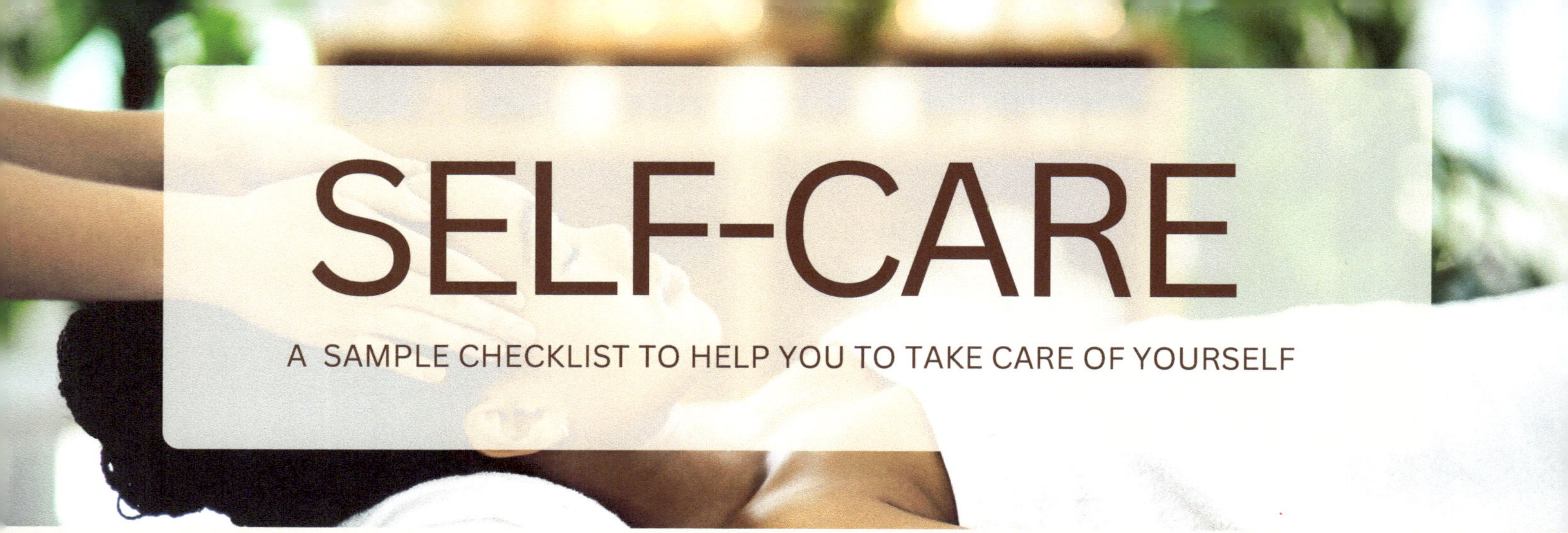

SELF-CARE

A SAMPLE CHECKLIST TO HELP YOU TO TAKE CARE OF YOURSELF

Tasks	Sun	Mon	Tue	Wed	Thu	Fri	Sat
Meditate/Prayer	●	●	●	●	●	●	●
Morning Yoga	●	●	●	●	●	●	●
Eat Veggies with Every Meal	●	●	●	●	●	●	●
Drink enough Water	●	●	●	●	●	●	●
Daily Gratitude Practice	●	●	●	●	●	●	●
Walk in an enjoyable environment	●	●	●	●	●	●	●
Sit in Sunlight	●	●	●	●	●	●	●

PROTECT THE WAY YOU DIGEST

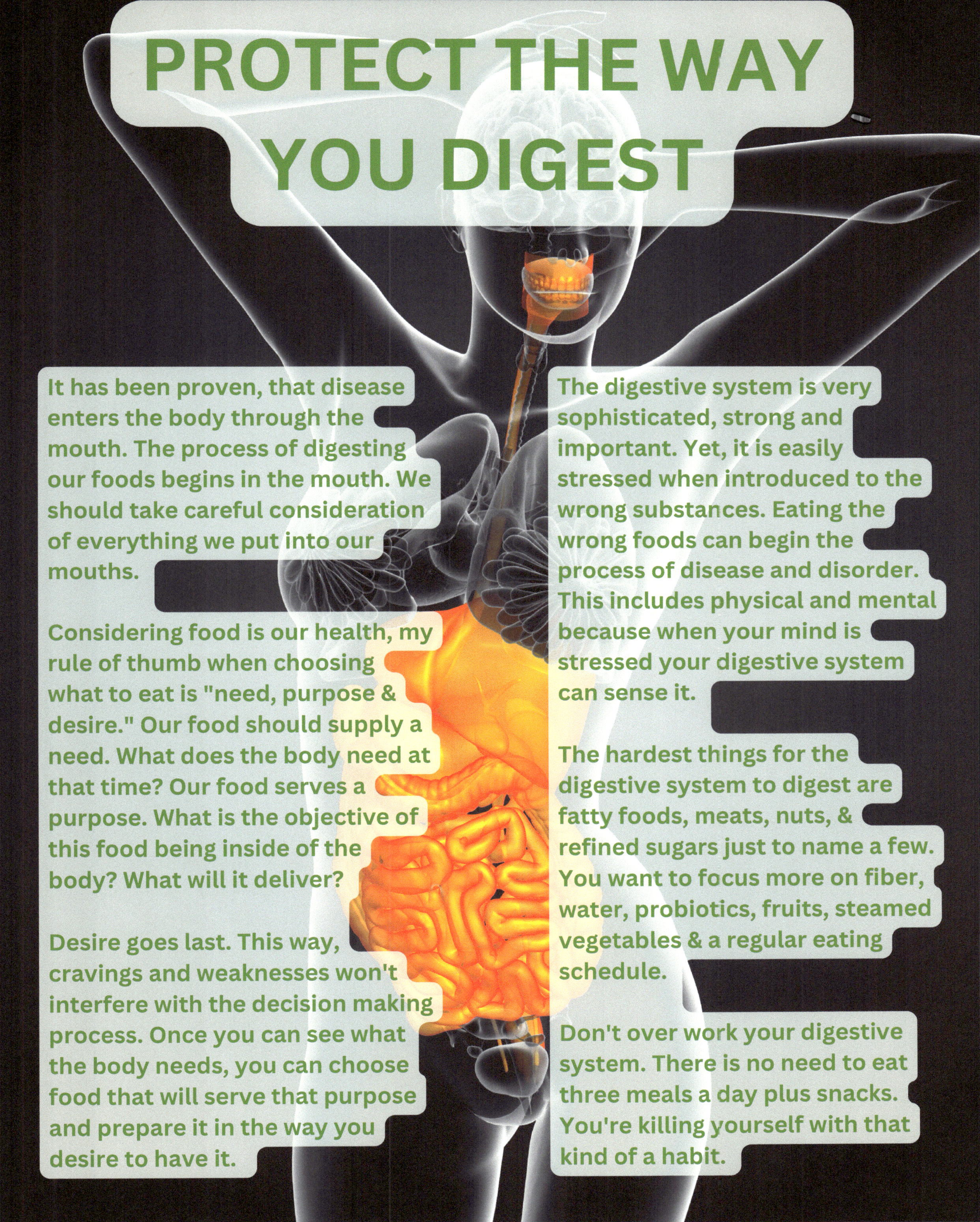

It has been proven, that disease enters the body through the mouth. The process of digesting our foods begins in the mouth. We should take careful consideration of everything we put into our mouths.

Considering food is our health, my rule of thumb when choosing what to eat is "need, purpose & desire." Our food should supply a need. What does the body need at that time? Our food serves a purpose. What is the objective of this food being inside of the body? What will it deliver?

Desire goes last. This way, cravings and weaknesses won't interfere with the decision making process. Once you can see what the body needs, you can choose food that will serve that purpose and prepare it in the way you desire to have it.

The digestive system is very sophisticated, strong and important. Yet, it is easily stressed when introduced to the wrong substances. Eating the wrong foods can begin the process of disease and disorder. This includes physical and mental because when your mind is stressed your digestive system can sense it.

The hardest things for the digestive system to digest are fatty foods, meats, nuts, & refined sugars just to name a few. You want to focus more on fiber, water, probiotics, fruits, steamed vegetables & a regular eating schedule.

Don't over work your digestive system. There is no need to eat three meals a day plus snacks. You're killing yourself with that kind of a habit.

MYTH OR FACTS

ABOUT DIGESTION

Raw vegetables are better for the digestive system.

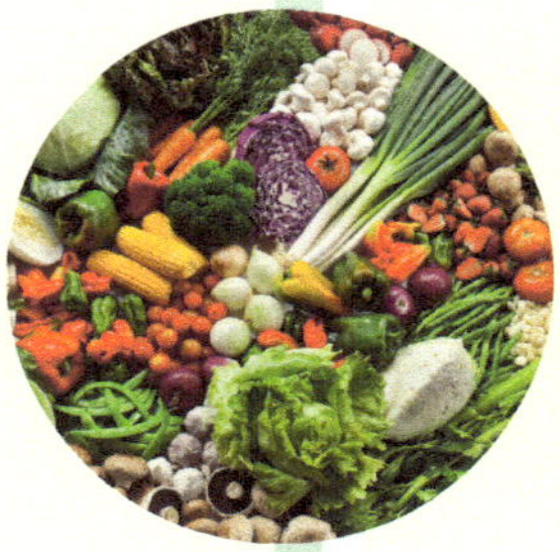

Cooking vegetables breaks down some of its fibers and cell walls making it easier to digest.

Spicy foods cause ulcers.

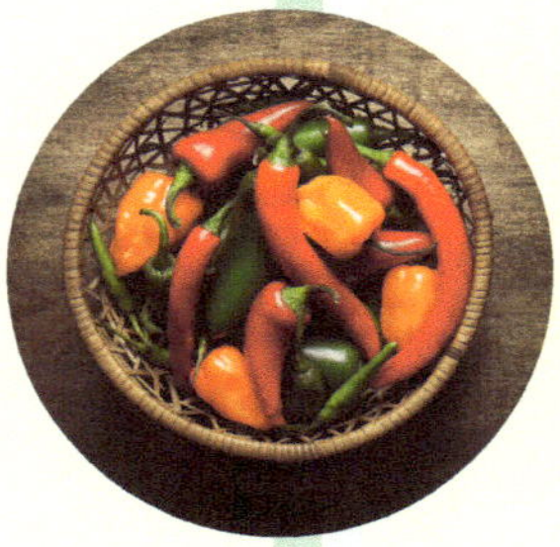

Spicy foods do not cause ulcers. They may lead to stomachaches for some but they have been proven to not cause ulcers.

Kale is a healthy vegetable to eat.

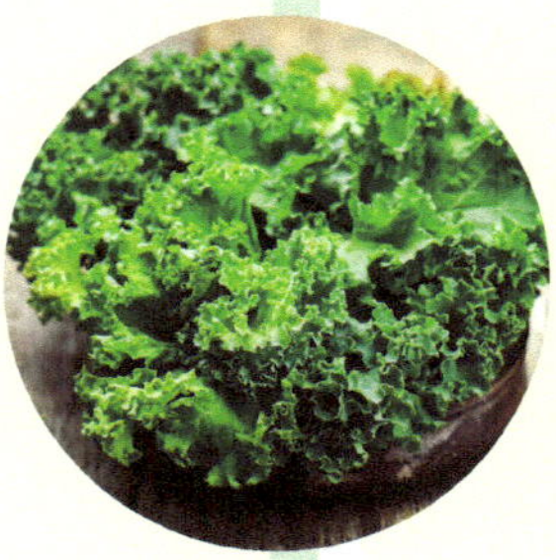

Kale contains fructans & galactans which are difficult to digest & some times impossible. This puts stress on the digestive system.

Nuts are a great snack. Our digestive system loves them.

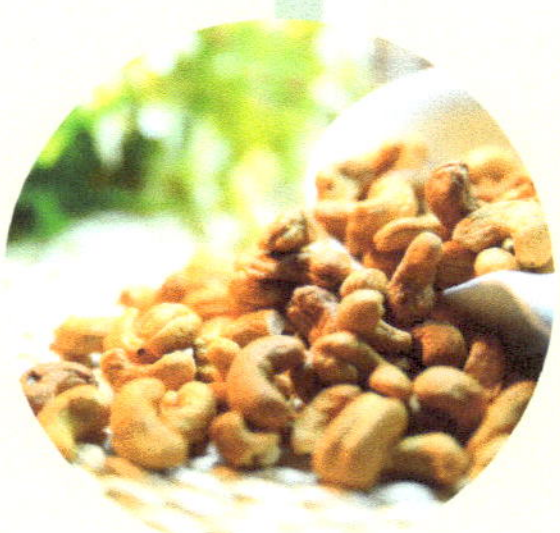

Nuts contain high fats & fiber making them hard to digest. Fiber is a carbohydrate that our bodies can not digest at all.

MOST COMMON MISTAKES MADE WITH DIGESTION

NOT DRINKING ENOUGH WATER

Gut health is not all about food, it also includes the fluids we drink. Water is very important to drink. It helps to prevent constipation, it lubricates your joints, helps the kidneys and liver to flush toxins out of the body & more!

EATING TOO FAST

Take your time and chew your food. Remember digestion begins in the mouth. The more you chew your food the less the stomach has to do. We don't want our stomachs to wear out too fast and begin to cause digestive issues or create ulcers.

OVER EATING

There are only so many digestive enzymes available at a time. The more food you eat, the longer it takes to digest the food. When you create a habit of over eating, food builds up and will remain in the stomach too long which creates fat.

DRINKING TOO MUCH CAFFINATED BEVERAGES

Too much caffine can lead to diarrhea & the overproduction of stomach acidity. Too much caffeine may also damage the liver, causing the inability to control urine & create restlessness. Drinking one cup of coffee in the morning is fine, but 4 cups or more a day is excessive.

TOP FIVE FOODS THAT CAUSE INFLAMMATION

A build up of inflammation in the body can cause diseases like diabetes, high blood pressure, cancer, liver or kidney disease.

01

FRIED FOODS

Fried foods have tons of trans fats in them which trigger inflammation production in the body. Fried foods also cause damage to the gut microbiome, which puts you at a higher risk for some diseases.

02

RED MEATS

Red meats raise the levels of oxidative stress, which leads to the production of inflammation. Oxidative stress interferes with the detoxification process of the foods we eat.

03

REFINED GRAINS

Refined grains include white rice, white bread, pasta, and breakfast cereals. The process that grains go through to become refined causes inflammation and a spike in blood sugar levels.

04

SODAS/POP

The high sugar content in soda/pop causes the production of inflammation in the body. This may come as a surprise but, even diet and so called sugar-free sodas cause inflammation.

05

SNACK FOODS/REFINED SUGAR

Snack foods that fall into this category are foods like cookies, chips, cakes, crackers & pastries. Unnatural sugars stimulates the production of fatty acids in your liver which triggers the production of inflammation in the body.

STRONG NATURAL ANTI-INFLAMMATORY FOODS

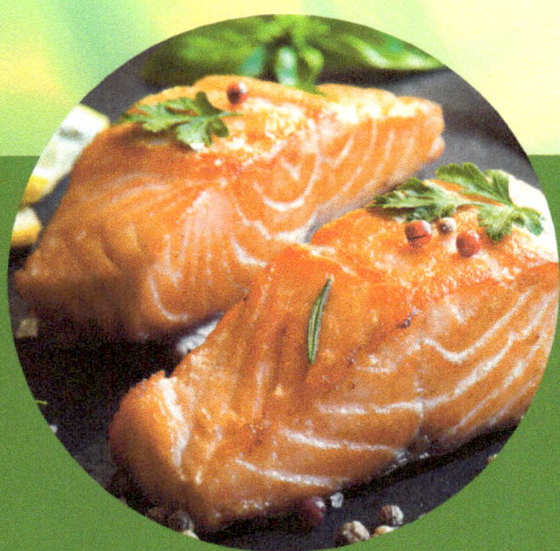

Salmon

Omega-3 Fatty Acids

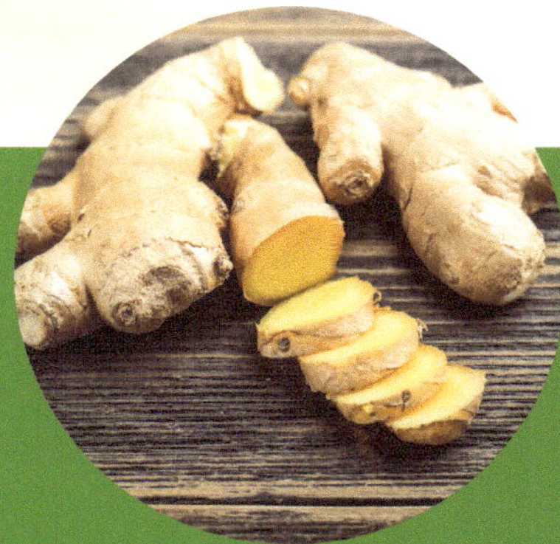

Ginger

Spice or Herb

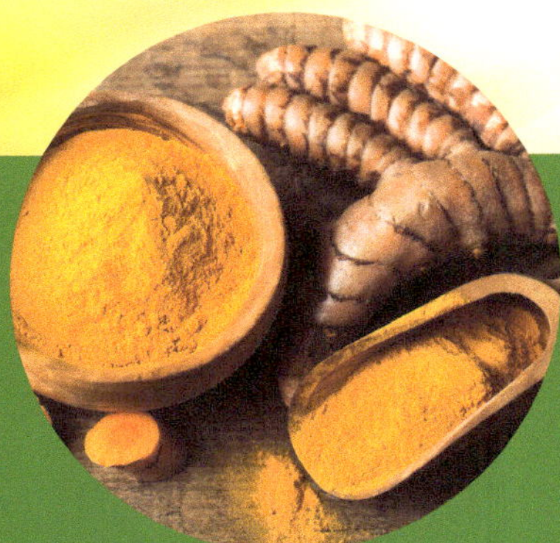

Turmeric

Spice or Herb

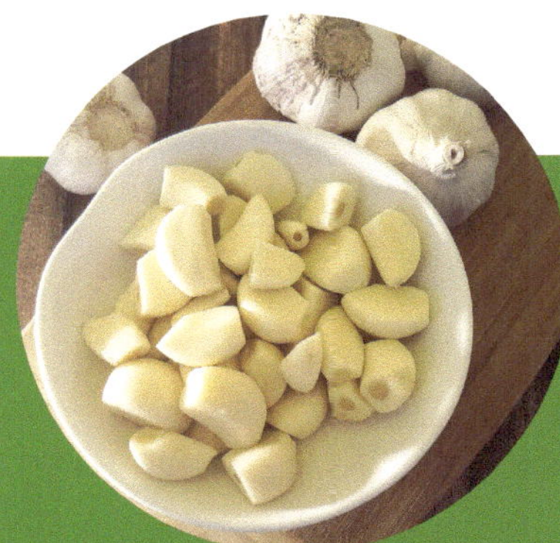

Garlic

Spice or Vegetable

NO SUCH THING AS A NO CARB DIET!

First let's be clear, carbohydrates are one of the MAIN nutrients in your food that is going to provide energy for your body. The question is, what carbs are ok for your lifestyle vs the heavy carbs that may not match or compliment your daily activity. This is the area people usually misunderstand which can lead to weight gain, sluggish feelings, heart disease, bloating and even high blood sugar levels.

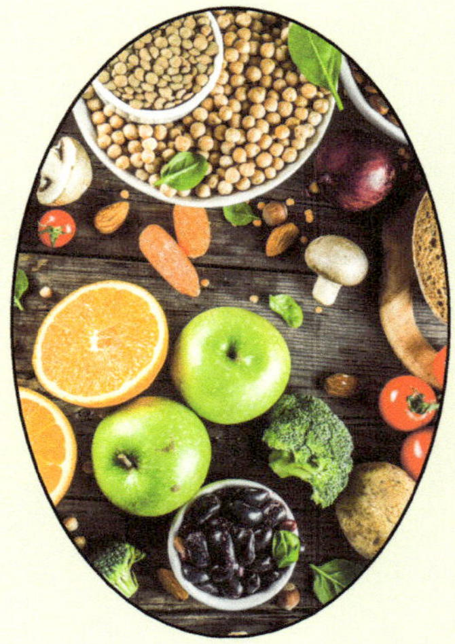

Carbohydrates are found in a category of either simple or complex. Simple carbs are bad carbs found in white sugar, pasta, white flour, white rice and some cereals to name a few. Simple carbs are carbohydrates that have been stripped of fiber, nutrients and bran. What purpose does it serve to eat a food substance that is not giving your body what it needs to function properly?

Complex carbohydrates are what you want in your diet, with the proper balance of intake that matches your daily activity. Let's take a snap shot at what that looks like, keeping in mind ALL foods have a form of carbohydrates in them.

QUICK TIP

Eat more fiber rich fruits and vegetables.
Limit or eliminate foods and juices with added sugars.

DO YOU HAVE A SEDENTARY LIFESTYLE?

TEST YOURSELF

1 How long do you sit everyday?

- More than 60 minutes at a time
- 30-45 minutes at a time
- Move around the majority of the day

2 In the course of your day, how many hours are you actually moving around?

- 1-2 hours
- 3-4 hours
- More than 4 hours

3 How often do you feel tired?

- When you first wake up in the morning?
- All thoughout your day
- Only when your day is completed, if then.

4 Have you gained any weight in the last 3-6 months unintentionally?

- Yes, but no more than 5 pounds
- Yes, 10-20 pounds
- No

5 Is your memory cloudy?

- Yes, everyday
- Yes, but not often
- Not at all

6 Do you suffer from anxiety or depression?

- Yes, all the time
- Yes, sometimes
- No, not at all

WHICH CARBS SHOULD BE IN YOUR DIET

1. The Sedentary lifestyle

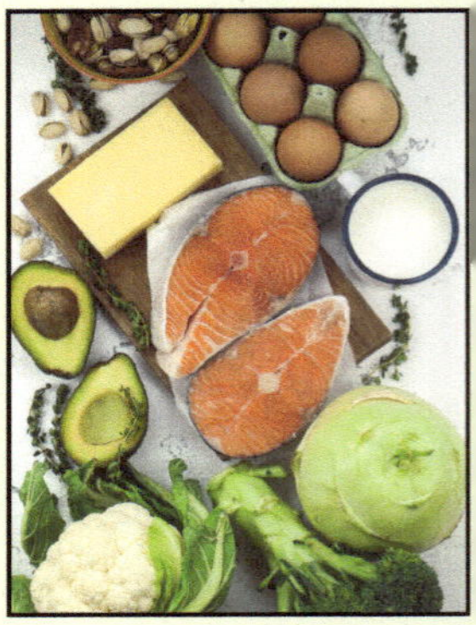

If you are sitting most of the day, meaning you take fewer than 5,000 steps a day and have a low laborious job, you need to stick to the diet that compliments the sedentary lifestyle. This consists of foods in the low carbohydrate category of unsaturated fats like plant based proteins (beans & lentils), fruits, vegetables, eggs, seafood and whole wheat toast.

Stay away from starches like white rich, potatoes, pasta, fried foods and fast food. They are not your friends.

2. The Moderate lifestyle

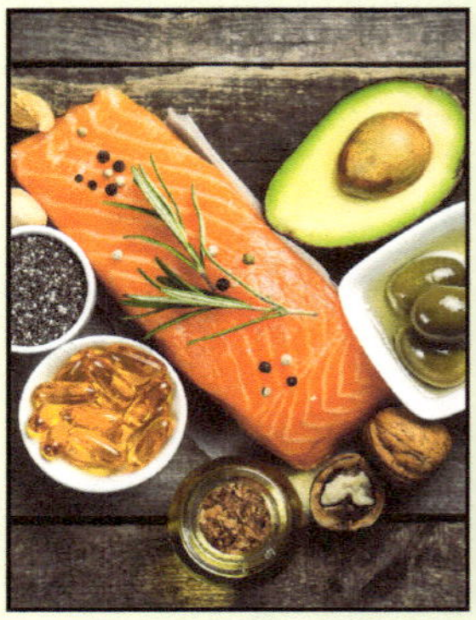

With the moderate lifestyles you are taking 7,500 - 10,000 steps per day and you are averaging 30-60 minutes of physical activity per day that increases the heart rate and causes the body to sweat. This type of lifestyle can stick to the low carbs foods with unsaturated fats too. You can only afford to put a little bit more on your plate than the sedentary lifestyle and you get a dessert treat day once every other week. The Key is to stay healthy!

3. The Active Lifestyle

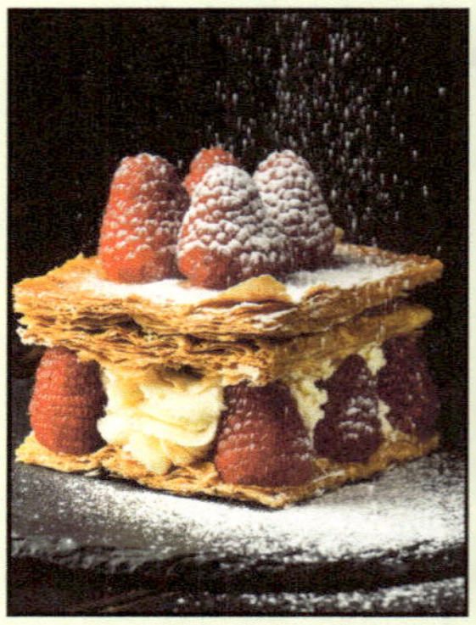

If you are averaging more than 60 minutes of activity per day and you're averaging 10,000 - 23,000 steps per day, you belong in this lifestyle section. You've earned your cheat day with your favorite dessert! Occasionally, you can have pasta, pizza or even potatoes. Not too often though, occasionally can be once a week or once every other week. Keep in mind, regardless of your lifestyle category you still want to eat healthy foods.

LOW CARBS SHOPPING LIST

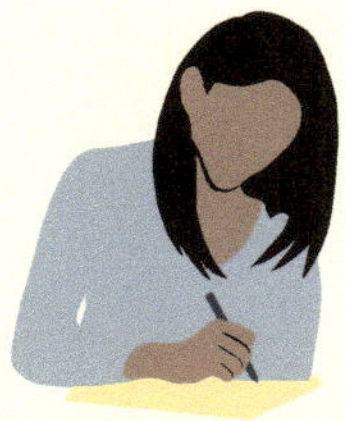
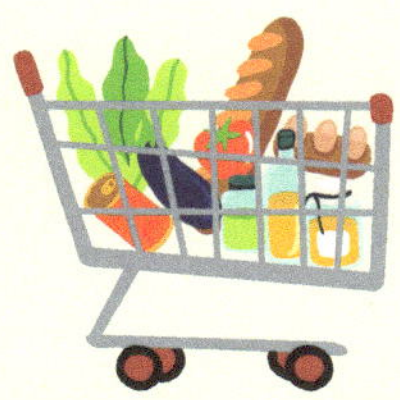
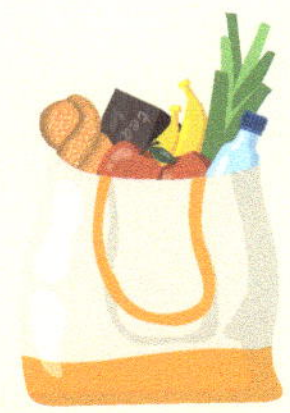

ITEM	CATEGORY
LETTUCE	Vegetable
AVOCADOS	Fruit
GREEN BEANS	Vegetable
TOMATOES	Fruit
ZUCHINNI	Vegetable
PEPPERS	Fruit
EGGPLANT	Fruit
GARLIC	Vegetable/ Allium
ONIONS	Vegetable/ Allium
BERRIES (STRAWBERRIES, BLUE BERRIES, RASPBERRIES, ETC)	Fruit
CANTALOUPE	Fruit
EGGS	Protein
WHOLE MILK	Dairy
BEANS (SMALL NAVY OR BLACK BEANS)	Legume
OILS (OLIVE OIL, GRAPESEED OIL, ETC)	Unsaturated Fats
GRASS FED LAMB OR BEEF	Meats/Protein
GUACAMOLE	Fruit
HERBAL SPICES	Botanical
SALMON	Fish
STUFFED BLACK OLIVES	Stone Fruits

*This list is a sample list to help guide you on how to create your own.

Proper Food Portions

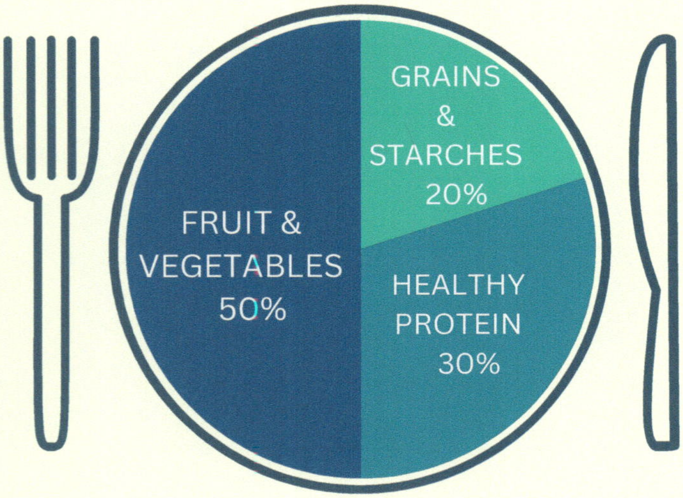

Sedentary Lifestyle

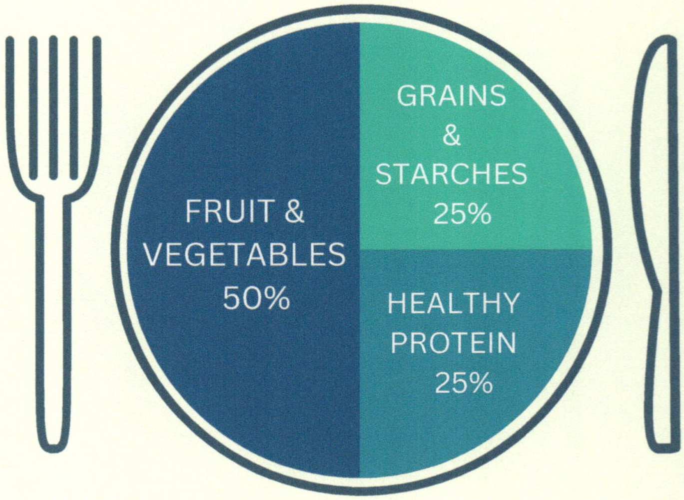

Moderate Lifestyle

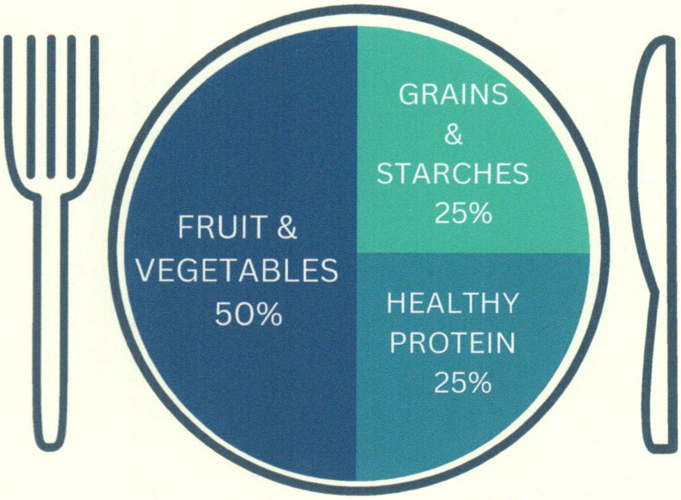

Active Lifestyle

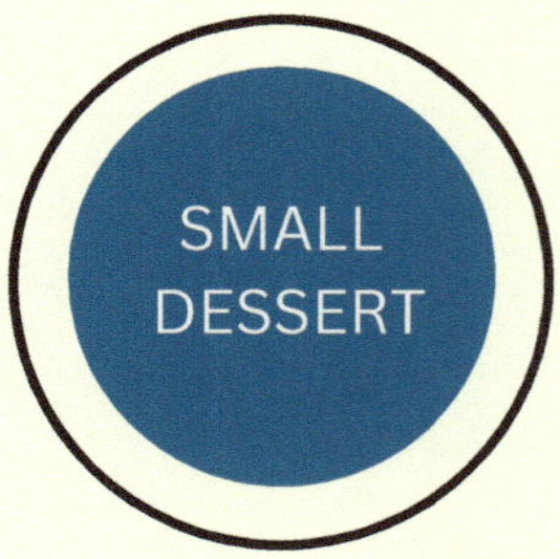

Once a week Treat Day

For Everyone

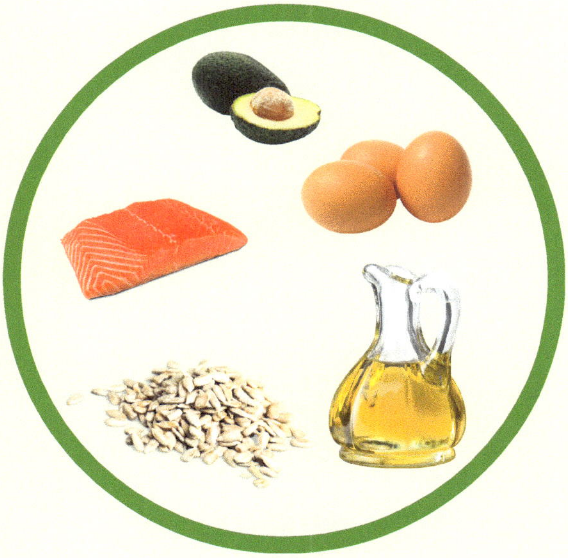

Unsaturated Fats
&
Oils

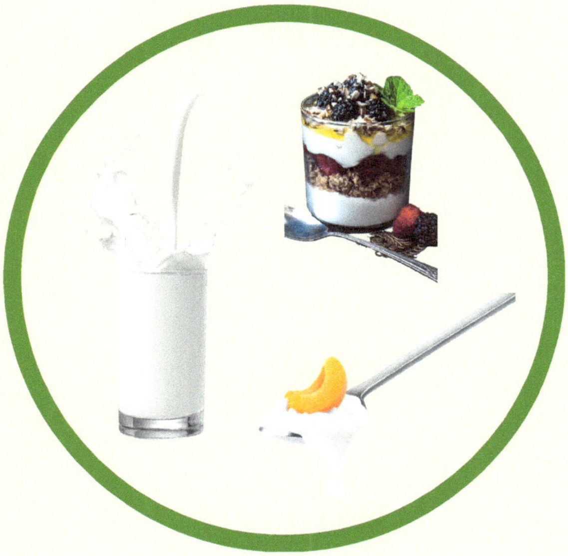

Dairy

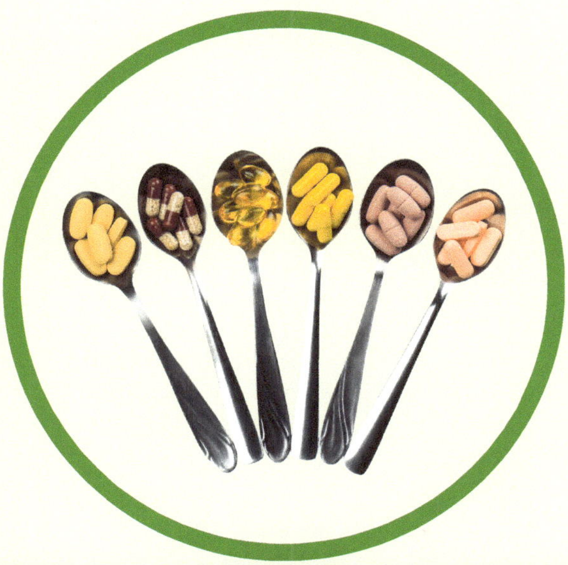

Supplements

Weekly Healthy Meal Plan

Date :

YOU DON'T NEED 3 MEALS A DAY AND 2 SNACKS!

Monday

Tuesday

Wednesday

Thursday

Friday

Saturday

Sunday

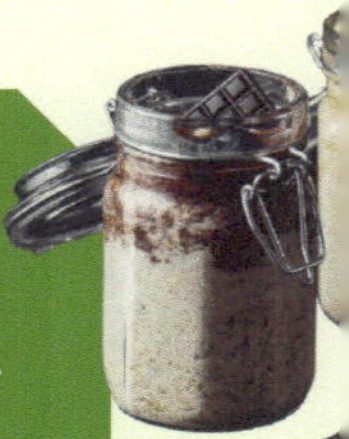

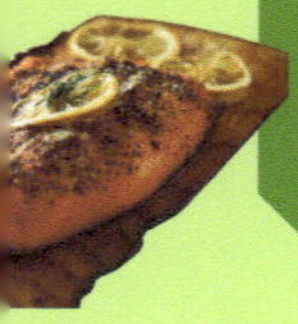

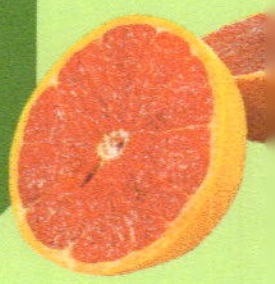

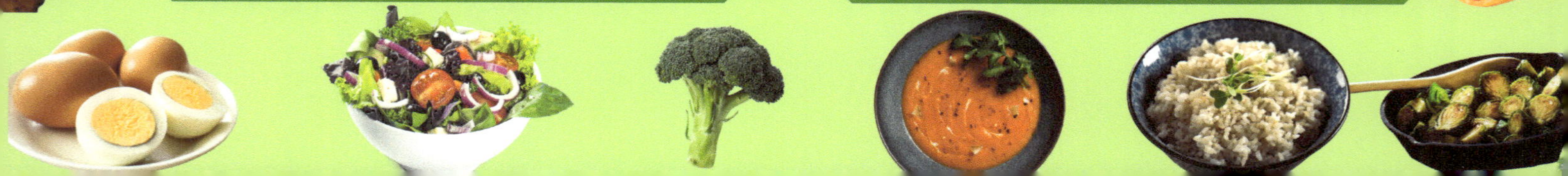

WATER BALANCE

Water is one of life's essential needs, we can not live sufficiently without it. Water balance in the body is described as matching the amount of water you take in daily with the amount of water you lose daily. Determining how much water you need daily includes factoring in your weight, gender, activity level & what you eat. Not everyone needs eight glasses of water per day. Some need more and some need less.

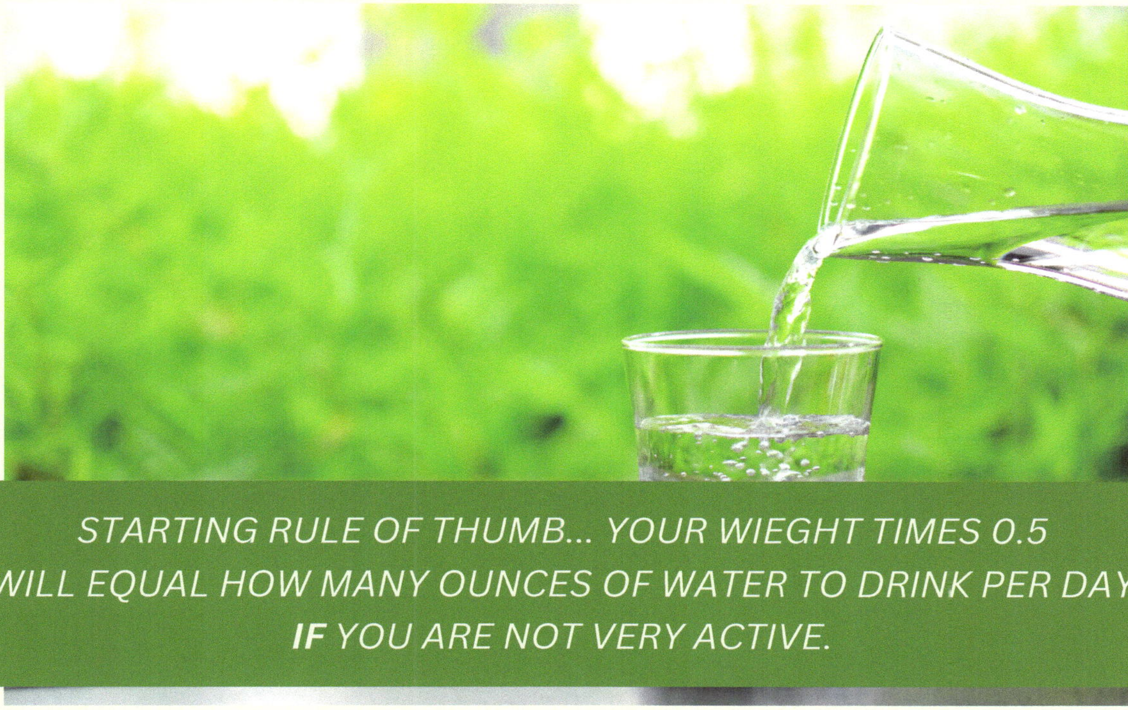

STARTING RULE OF THUMB... YOUR WIEGHT TIMES 0.5 WILL EQUAL HOW MANY OUNCES OF WATER TO DRINK PER DAY ***IF*** *YOU ARE NOT VERY ACTIVE.*

5 FACTS ABOUT WATER

1

Your body as a whole is 75% water. You brain & heart by itself is about 73% water. Your lungs are about 83% water and your skin contains about 64% water.

2

Water carries nutrients & oxygen to the cells of your body. It is the main property of blood. Water helps convert food into energy.

3

Water serves as a protector for organs and tissues of the body. It even protects your spinal cord, and lessens the burden on the kidney's & the liver.

4

Water helps your brain cells communicate with one another. It clears out toxins and waste that impairs brain function.

5

A small 2% decrease in hydration can result in short term memory loss. Inadequate water intake can cause abdominal pains & constipation.

WEEKLY FOOD LOG

BECOMING MORE MINDFUL OF WHAT YOU EAT!

WEEK OF :

	MON	TUE	WED	THU	FRI	SAT	SUN
DATE							
FOOD							
EXERCISE							
SNACKS							
WATER							

CLEANSE YOUR BODY FOR A FULL CYCLE OF REGENERATION

BALANCE YOUR WHEEL OF HEALTH

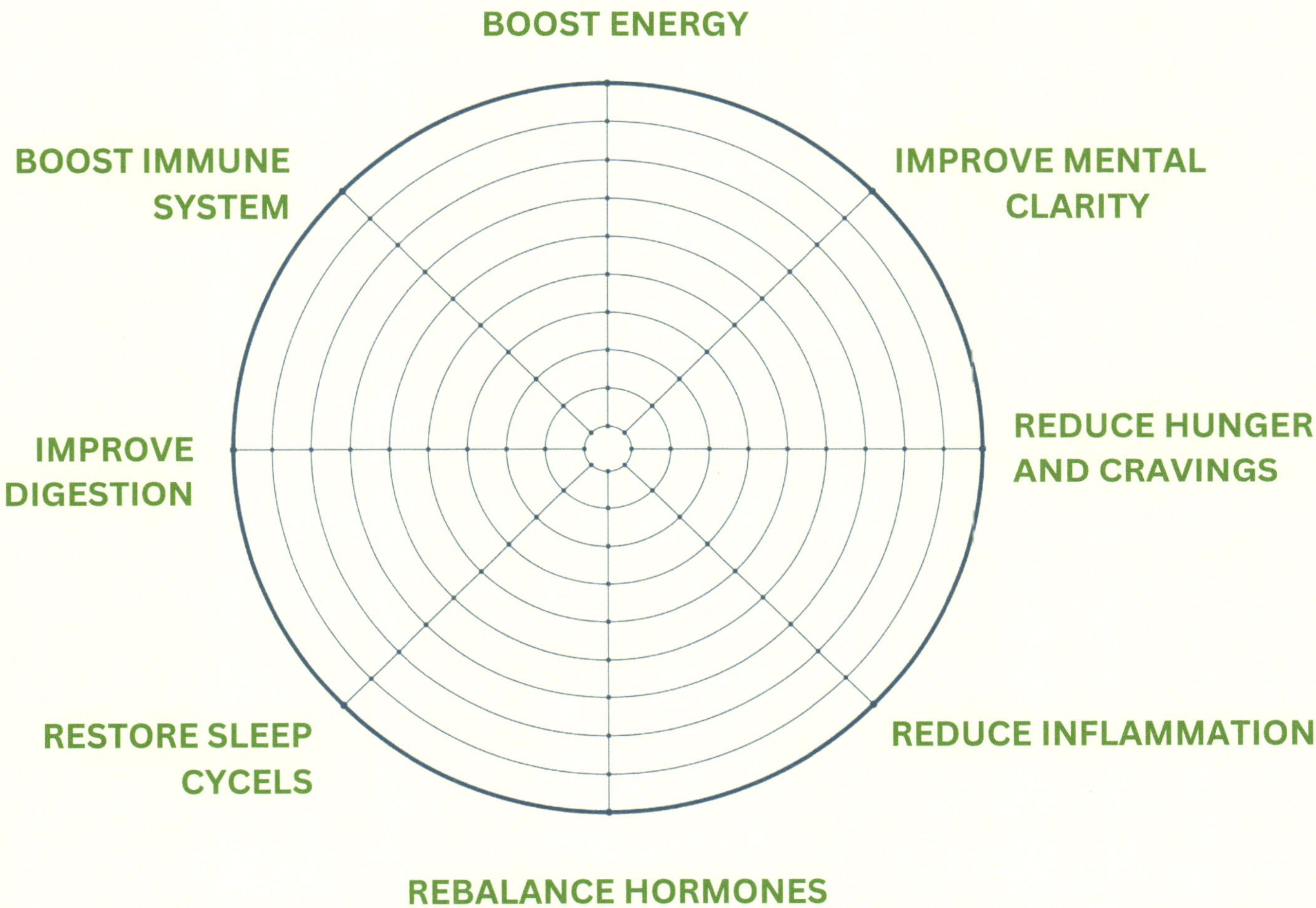

NEED SOME CLEANSING RECIPES?
LET'S GO!

WHY CLEANSE?

Some people cleanse as a weight loss program. Weight loss should never be the goal. Cleansing your body helps to reset the systems of the body. It removes unwanted toxins and bacteria. Cleansing can help with improving mental clarity, boosting your energy, taking away food cravings and hunger, restore sleep cycles, balance hormones and so much more! Don't cheapen yourself with the weight loss goal. Know that you are worth the healthy lifestyle changing goal, which will lead to the unwanted weight falling off . This is the type of goal that doesn't change back but instead transforms your existence!

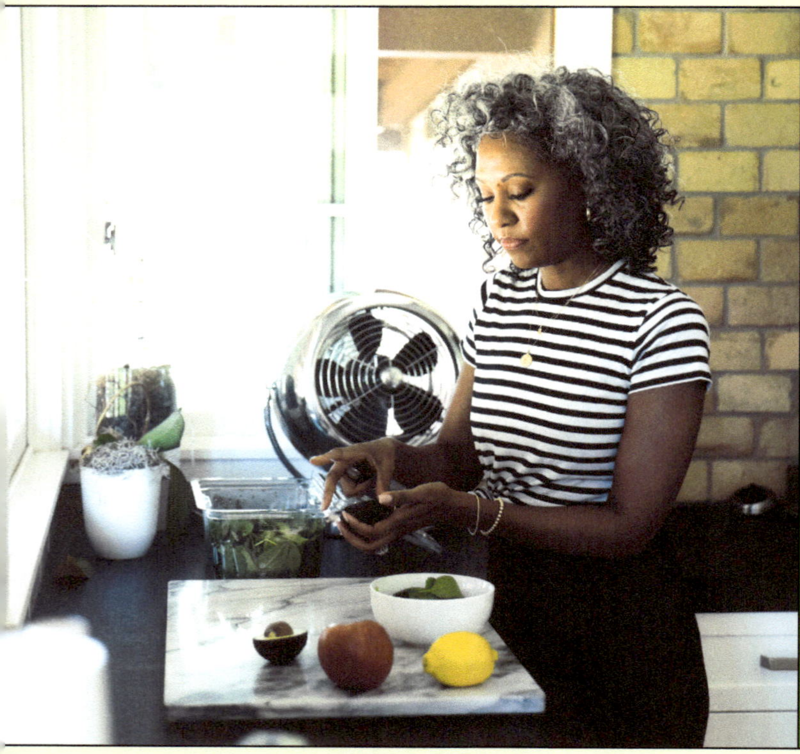

✦ QUICK TIP ✦

- Add probiotics to your diet when on a cleanse
- Drink plenty of water
- Sweat Regularly
- Fast Regularly
- Get Quality Sleep

THERE ARE MANY TYPES OF BODY CLEANSES & DETOX'S

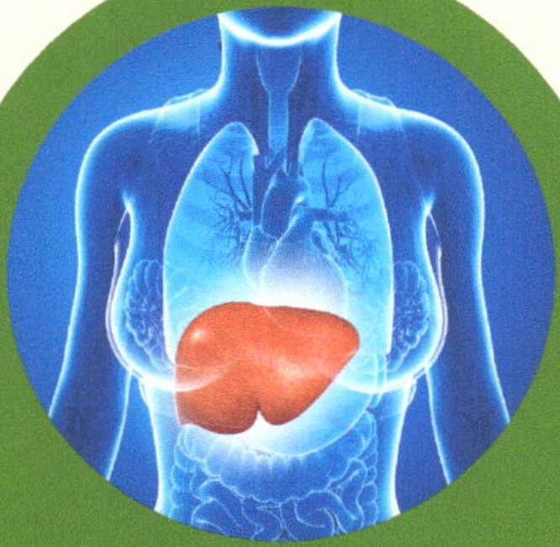

DETOX

A detox of your body is not the same as a body cleanse, eventhough they both center around clean healthy foods. When you detox your body you're focusing on removing toxins from the body. You are giving your liver a chance to reboot itself & the room it needs to start processing toxins again.

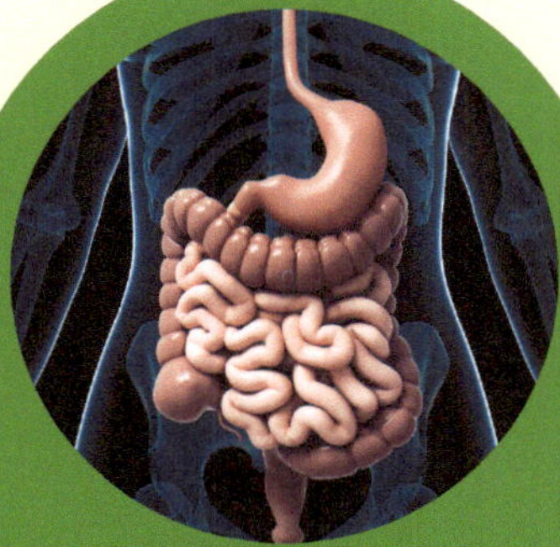

CLEANSE

When you want to focus on the overall health of your digestive system, you want to do a cleanse.

Cleanses are known to help fight bloating & incorporate regular bowel movements. They are also an excellent way to maintain your health in-between or after a detox.

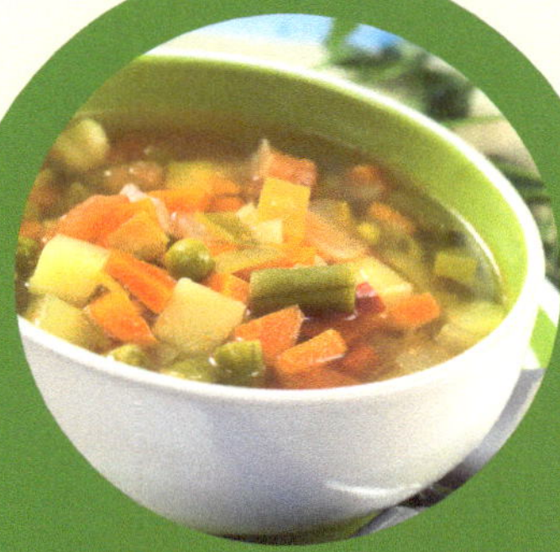

SOUPING

Souping is a very healthy type of cleanse. You can do it for one day or multiple days. In comparison to juicing, soup is low in sugar and can be loaded with fiber making it more filling.

Soups are loaded with minerals, vitamins, antioxidants & are easily digested.

!

In preparing your body for a cleanse or detox you want to stay away from alcohol, processed foods, excess levels of caffeine, red meats and sugars. Always consult with a doctor before doing a detox or cleanse, if you have any diseases, illnesses, are pregnant or lactating.

SYMPTOMS Q&A

If you answer yes to any of these questions or symptoms, your body needs to detox or cleanse.

DO YOU CARRY UNWANTED WEIGHT?	○ - YES	○ - NO
DO YOU HAVE ANY FOOD INTOLERANCES?	○ - YES	○ - NO

HOW OFTEN DO YOU EXPERIENCE ANY OF THE FOLLOWING SYMPTOMS?

	NEVER	1-2 /MONTH	3-4 /MONTH	1-3 /WEEK	EVERY DAY
CONSTIPATION	○	○	○	○	○
UPSET STOMACH	○	○	○	○	○
ABDOMINAL PAIN	○	○	○	○	○
HEARTBURN	○	○	○	○	○
BLOATING	○	○	○	○	○
ANXIETY	○	○	○	○	○
INSOMNIA	○	○	○	○	○
FATIGUE	○	○	○	○	○
BODY ACHES	○	○	○	○	○
ARTHRITIS	○	○	○	○	○
GOUT	○	○	○	○	○
MEMORY ISSUES	○	○	○	○	○
BRAIN FOG	○	○	○	○	○
SINUS PROBLEMS	○	○	○	○	○
ACNE / SKIN ISSUES	○	○	○	○	○

DETOX SYMPTOMS THAT MAY OCCUR

SYMPTOM	SUGGESTION
CONSTIPATION	Try drinking more water and incorporating more fiber into your diet.
UPSET STOMACH	Definitely drink more water and rest. Just remember to stick with the process. Your body is removing toxins.
GROWLING STOMACH	One thing you can do is slow down while eating. Swallow your food before opening your mouth for another bite.
HUNGER	Try drinking herbal teas.
HEADACHE	Headaches during a detox is usually related to dehydration. Drink water and decaffeinated tea.
FEELING LIGHT HEADED	Stop the detox if this lasts beyond minutes or is accompanied by shortness of breathe & inform your doctor.
FEELING COLD	This is normal. As your body detoxifies, the inflammation is cooling down.
NAUSIA	This may occur when people are detoxifying from alcohol, drugs or sugar. It's normal. Just stay hydrated.
FATIGUE	Give your body the rest it craves. Take naps. Your bodyis working to get the toxins out.
BRAIN FOG	Brain Fog is normal. Just stick with the process and know when it's over you should feel better.

YOUR CLEANSING NOTES

Being mindful of the process

DAY

01

WHAT SYMPTOMS ARE YOU EXPERIENCING TODAY?

DAY

02

WHAT SYMPTOMS ARE YOU EXPERIENCING TODAY?

DAY

03

WHAT SYMPTOMS ARE YOU EXPERIENCING TODAY?

POST CLEANSE

YES! YOU DID IT!
You are a woman of action that set her mind to cross the finish line & YOU WON!
CONGRATULATIONS!

Once you have finished your detox or cleanse you want to eat fruits and vegetables and continue to drink plenty of water on the first day and easy digestible foods for the next few days. You are easing yourself back into a normal, healthy routine. Regardless of how long you've cleansed for, you've just given your body a bit of a spring clean - it would be a shame to spoil this with overly processed foods, heavy animal produce or excessive amounts of sugar.

Reward yourself! YOU DID IT! Keep in mind, once you complete short healthy goals you have the ability & strength to make them permanent! It doesn't matter if you did a one day cleanse or a five day cleanse. What matters is you succeeded in reaching the goal even if you weren't perfect at achieving it! Enjoy the moment of such an accomplishment!

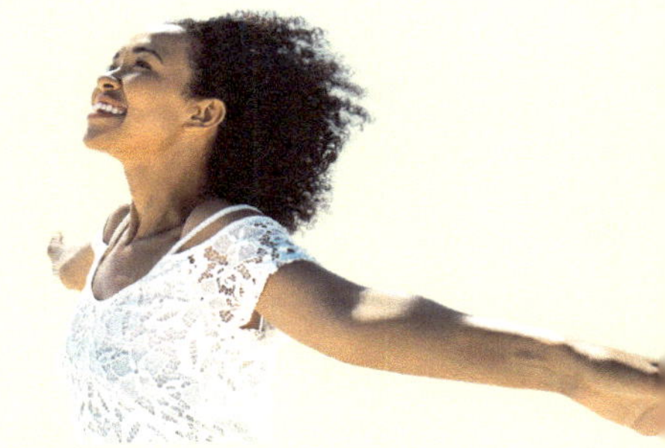

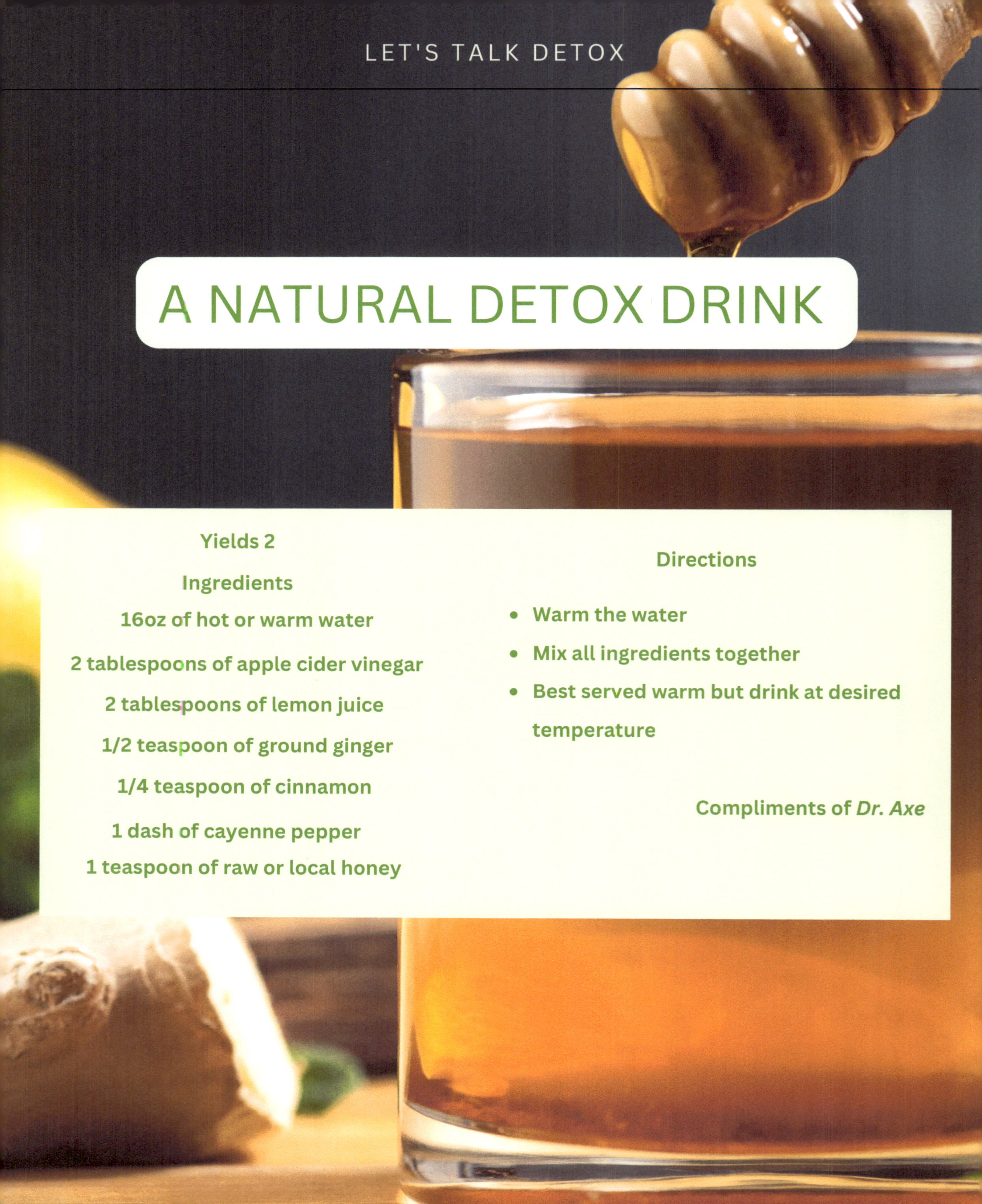

A NATURAL DETOX DRINK

Yields 2

Ingredients

16oz of hot or warm water

2 tablespoons of apple cider vinegar

2 tablespoons of lemon juice

1/2 teaspoon of ground ginger

1/4 teaspoon of cinnamon

1 dash of cayenne pepper

1 teaspoon of raw or local honey

Directions

- **Warm the water**
- **Mix all ingredients together**
- **Best served warm but drink at desired temperature**

Compliments of *Dr. Axe*

LIME MINT COOLER

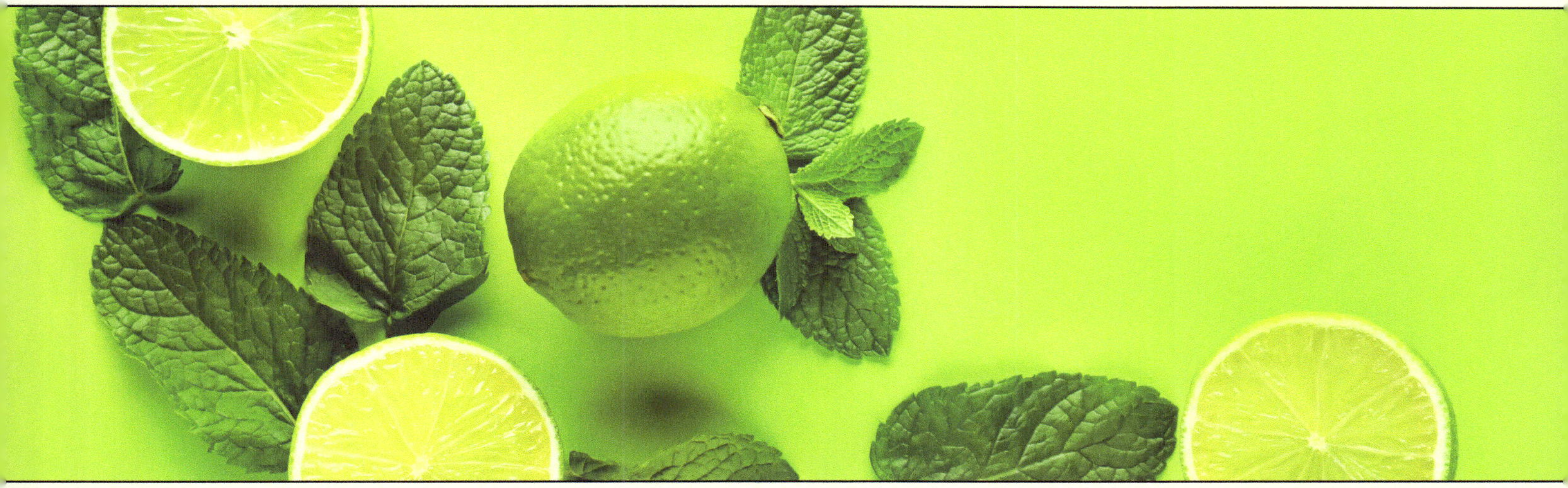

SERVES 1

FLUSHES TOXINS & IMPROVES SKIN TONE

Ingredients

5 or 6 fresh mint leaves

1 Lemon

1 tablespoon of honey/adjust to taste

1 tablespoon of ginger juice (optional)

2 cups of water

1 tablespoon of ice crushed

Directions

- Remove the seeds and extract the juice from the lemons and set aside.
- Place water, lime juice, ginger juice and honey into a blender and blend for a minute or so.
- Add mint leaves and let sit in the refrigerator for 30 min.
- Add crushed ice and enjoy!

WINTER DETOX ORANGE GINGER TURMERIC SMOOTHIE

Yields 2

Ingredients

2 navel oranges (quartered & peeled)

1 large carrot

1 inch piece of ginger

1 inch piece of turmeric peeled

(or 1 teaspoon of powdered turmeric)

A pinch of black pepper

Directions

- Add all the ingredients + 1 cup of ice cubes to your high-powered blender
- Blend on high until smooth. Add up to a cup of water for a more juice-like smoothie.

Compliments of *The Endless Meal*

IMMUNE BOOSTING ICE CUBES

Yields 12-24 ice cubes

Ingredients

2-3 large organic lemons

1/4 - 1/2 cups of spring water

Directions

- Add lemons to blender or food processor and blend.
- Slowly pour in the water a little at a time with the lemons for easier blending. Add more water as needed, but you don't want them watered down too much.
- Pour the blended lemons into ice cube trays & freeze.

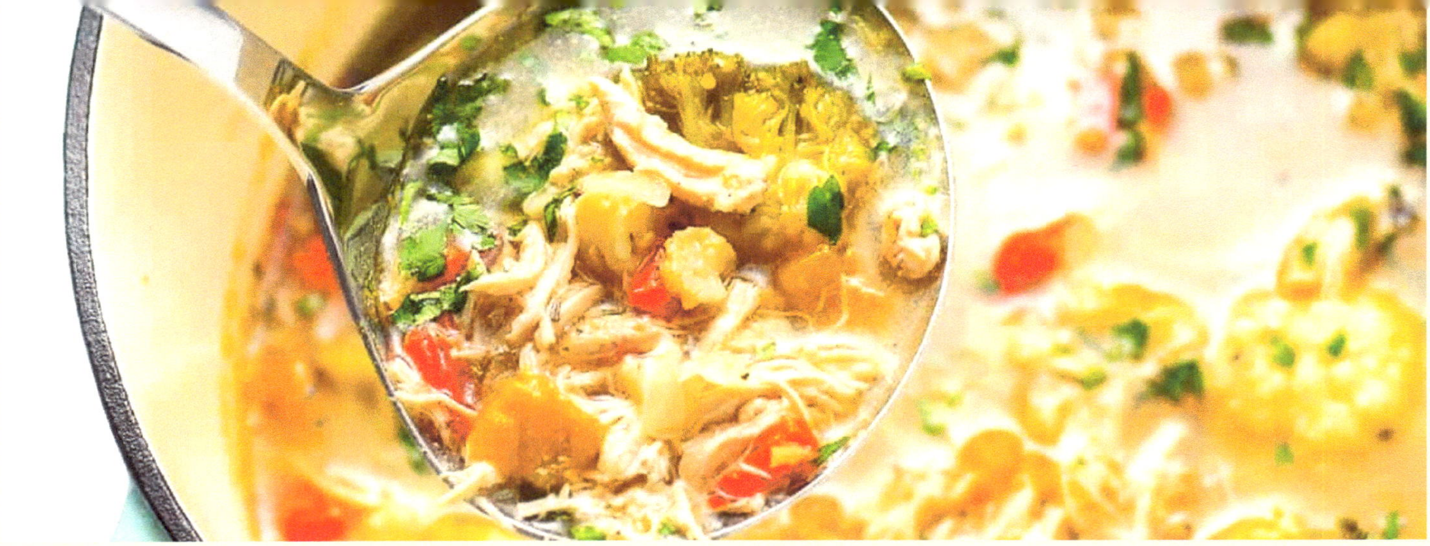

Healthy Detox Soup

SERVINGS: 6 | **PREPPING TIME: 14 MIN** | **COOKING TIME: 36 MIN**

Ingredients

2 tbsp Olive oil
1 medium Onion (diced)
3 cloves Garlic (minced)
1 tsp Fresh ginger (minced)
1/2 cup Bell peppers (diced)
1 tsp Italian seasoning (optional)
1/4 tsp Red pepper flakes (optional)
1 tsp Sea salt
1/2 tsp Black pepper
1 lb Boneless skinless chicken breasts
6 cups Chicken broth, reduced sodium
1 cup Broccoli (cut into florets)
1 cup Cauliflower (cut into florets)
2 tbsp Lemon juice

Directions

1. Heat the olive oil in a Dutch oven over medium-high heat.
2. Add the onion, garlic, and ginger saute for 3-4 minutes, until the garlic is fragrant and the onions are translucent
3. Add the bell peppers, Italian seasoning, red pepper flakes, sea salt, and black pepper. Cook for 3 more minutes.
4. Add the chicken breasts and chicken broth. Simmer for 20 minutes.
5. Remove the chicken breasts from the pot and shred using two forks. Add the shredded chicken back to the pot.
6. Add the broccoli and cauliflower florets. Simmer for 10 more minutes, until the cauliflower and broccoli are tender.
7. Remove from heat. Stir in the lemon juice

@Wholesomeyum.com By Maya Krampf

Healthy Habits Quiz

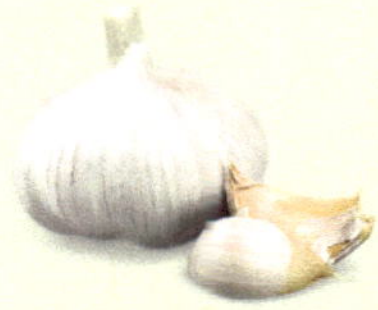

Applying what you have learned

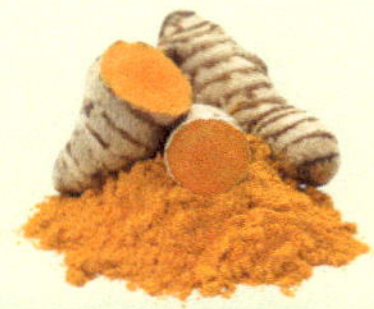

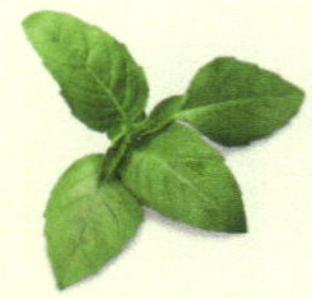

Answer the following questions to find out what you learned from this section

1. In understanding water balance, list three facts about water.

____

____

2. What should you eat if you're a diabetic? What should you avoid eating?

____

____

3. Knowing body movement is important, how much exercise should you do each day?

____

____

4. What are some items from the low carb shopping list?

____

____

5. What are some benefits of cleansing?

____

____

6. What should your proper food portions plate look like?

____

____

7. Why do you think it is important to keep your inner body clean?

____

Wellness Check In

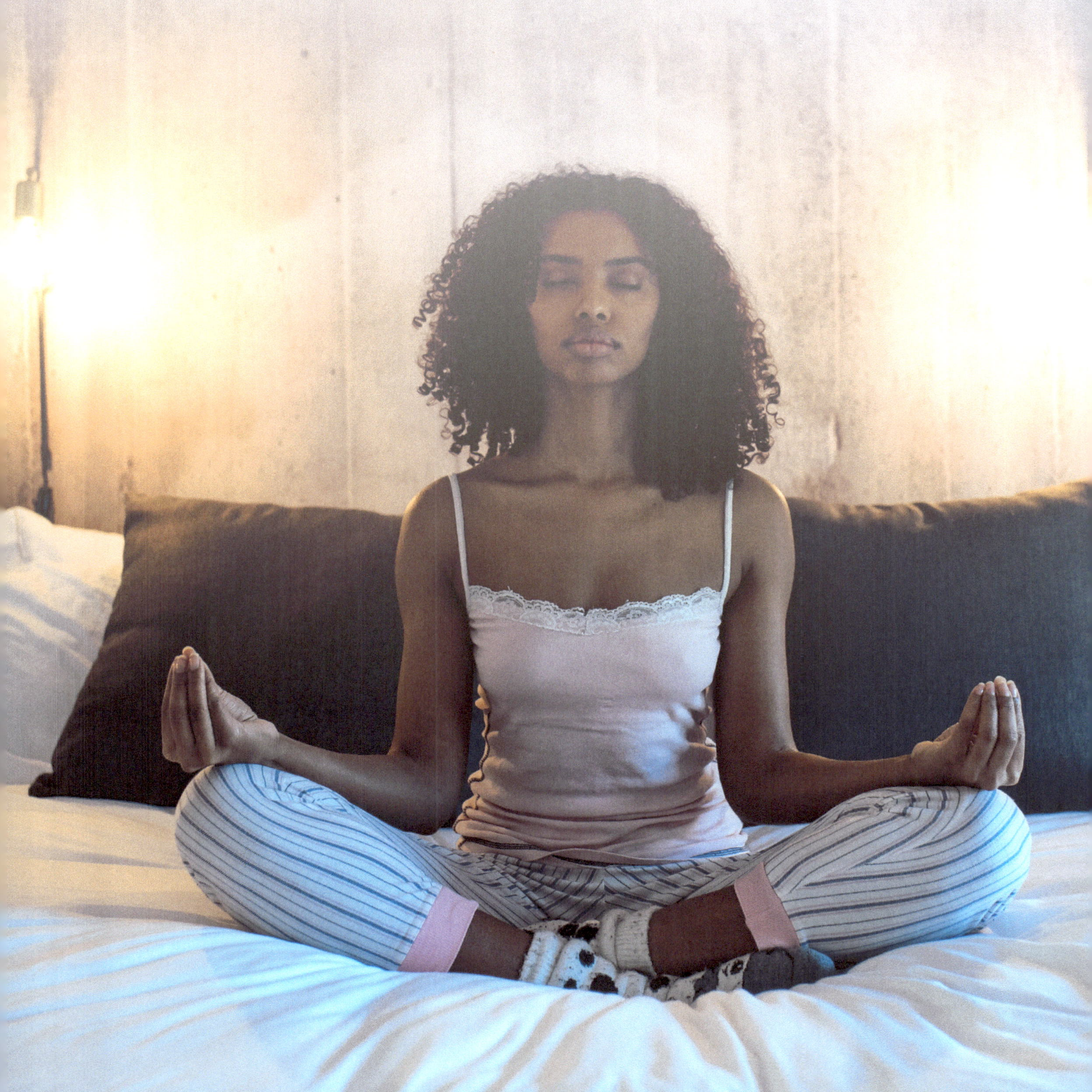

Release any triggers or uncomfortable feelings from this current chapter

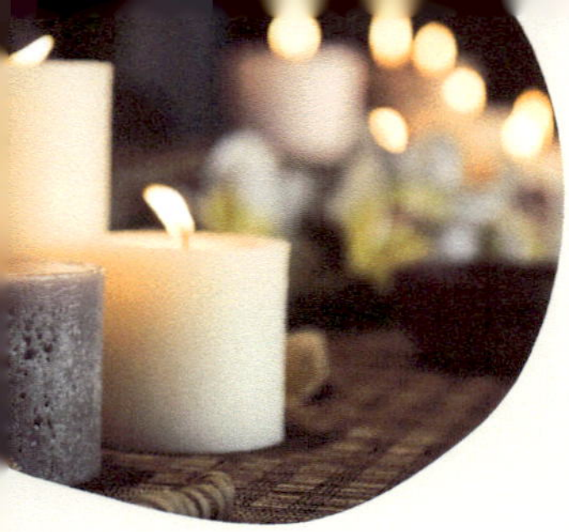

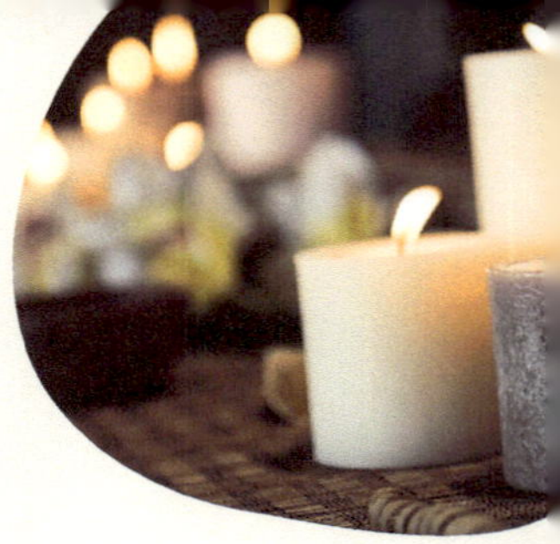

MINDFUL MEDITATION

FIVE MINUTE PROCESS

STEP ONE

SIT UP IN A CHAIR WITH YOUR BACK STRAIGHT. PLACE YOUR FEET FLAT ON THE FLOOR UNDER YOUR KNEES. REST THE PALMS OF YOUR HANDS ON YOUR THIGHS AND RELAX YOUR ARMS. LOOK STRAIGHT AHEAD BUT TRY NOT TO FOCUS ANYWHERE IN PARTICULAR. INSTEAD, NOTICE EVERYTHING IN THE ROOM AT ONCE. TAKE A DEEP BREATH AND START FEELING YOUR FEET. FEEL THEM TOUCHING THE FLOOR. FEEL YOUR FEET INTENSELY FROM THE INSIDE. DO NOT “THINK” ABOUT THEM, JUST FEEL THEM, SENSE THEM.

STEP TWO

AFTER A FEW BREATHS, MOVE YOUR ATTENTION TO YOUR CALVES. FEEL AND SENSE THEM FOR SEVERAL BREATHS. THEN MOVE YOUR ATTENTION FROM BODY PART TO BODY PART. FIRST TO YOUR THIGHS, THEN YOUR BOTTOM AGAINST THE CHAIR, TO YOUR ABDOMEN AND LOWER BACK, YOUR CHEST AND UPPER BACK, YOUR SHOULDERS, YOUR ARMS, YOUR HANDS, YOUR NECK, FACE, AND LASTLY YOUR HEAD. THEN LET YOUR AWARENESS COVER YOUR WHOLE BODY AT THE SAME TIME. THE IDEA IS TO “SCAN” YOUR BODY WITH YOUR ATTENTION, STOPPING FOR A FEW BREATHS ON EACH PART. THIS PRACTICE WILL STRENGTHEN YOUR ABILITY TO DIRECT AND HOLD YOUR ATTENTION.

STEP THREE

YOU MAY NOTICE THAT THE MOMENT YOU SIT DOWN, YOU START REMEMBERING THINGS AND FEEL THE URGE TO ACT ON THEM. THIS IS PART OF THE PROCESS. WHEN THOSE THOUGHTS COME AND TRY TO STEAL YOUR ATTENTION AWAY FROM YOUR BODY, SIMPLY SAY SILENTLY TO YOURSELF, “THANK YOU FOR SHARING,” AND DIRECT YOUR ATTENTION BACK TO YOUR BODY. BECOMING AWARE OF THIS UNDERLYING STATE IS THE FIRST STEP TOWARD DISSOLVING IT, AND CLAIMING BACK THE ENERGY IT CONSUMES.

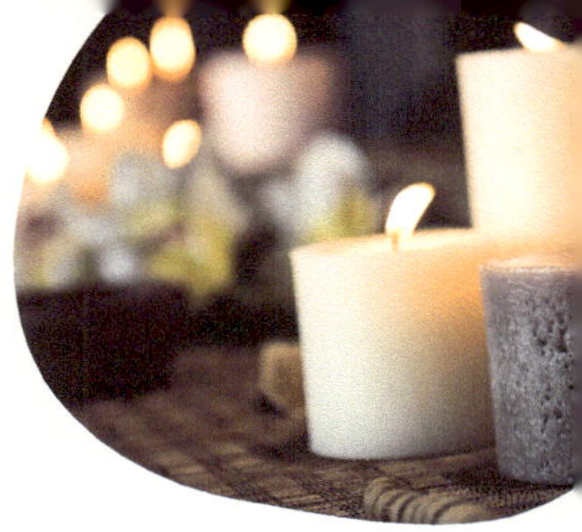

MINDFUL MEDITATION

FIVE MINUTE PROCESS

STEP FOUR

WHEN YOU FIND YOURSELF CONSUMED BY YOUR MIND, TRY FOR A SECOND TO SEPARATE YOUR ATTENTION FROM YOUR THOUGHTS AND RE-FOCUS IT ON THE PRESENT. THIS SMALL BOOST OF AWARENESS BREAKS THROUGH HABITUAL THOUGHT PATTERNS THAT LEAD AWAY FROM THE PRESENT MOMENT AND INTO DISTRACTED THOUGHTS. ANCHOR YOUR ATTENTION INTO THE PRESENT MOMENT AS OFTEN AS YOU CAN.

STEP FIVE

WHEN WE ARE NERVOUS, IT IS BECAUSE OUR UNCONSCIOUS THOUGHTS ARE INTERPRETING, JUDGING, MEASURING, AND EXPECTING. THIS UNCONCIOUS PROCESS CONSUMES VITAL ENERGY AND BUILDS ANXIETY. BY RE-DIRECTING OUR ATTENTION TO OUR BODY AND BREATH, WE RECLAIM THAT WASTED ENERGY. IT MAY BE HARD TO REMEMBER TO DO THIS IN DIFFICULT SITUATIONS. START WITH EASY ONES. BEGIN TO IMMEDIATELY SHIFT THE ENERGY OF ANY SITUATION.

STEP SIX

PRACTICING BEING PRESENT WILL HELP CLEAR OUT QUANTUM TOXINS FROM YOUR MIND. YOU WILL BEGIN TO BE ABLE TO USE YOUR ENERGY AND ATTENTION TO STAY PRESENT AND BE MORE PRODUCTIVE. THANK YOURSELF FOR COMPLETING THIS PROCESS!

This Weeks Self-care Plan

My Schedule

Mindful Meditation

My Top Priorities

Self

Note To Self

Daily Nutrition

Vegetable	
Fruit	
Protein	
Liquid	

STAGE ONE

Cholesterol LDL vs HDL

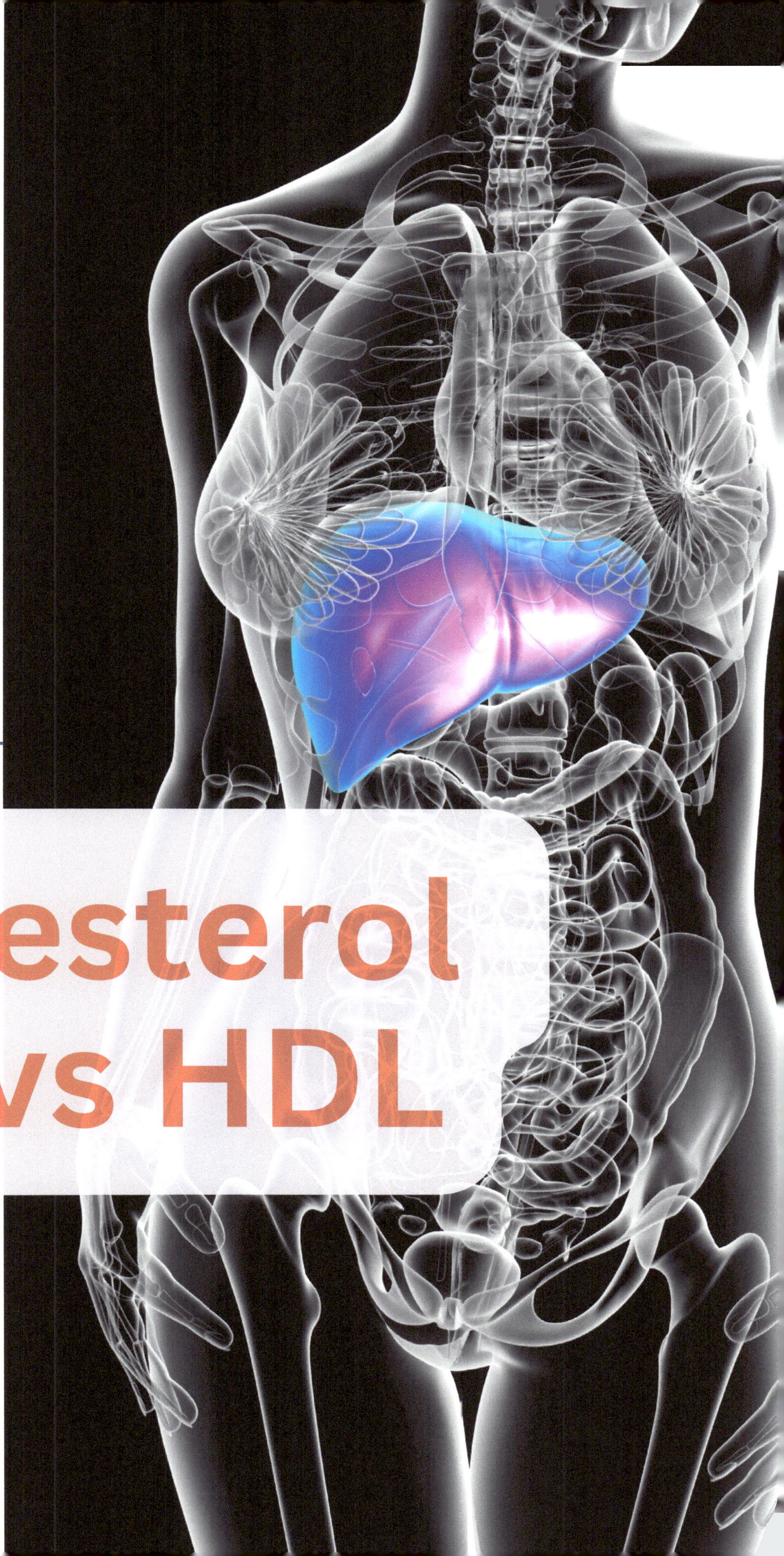

WHERE IS CHOLESTEROL PRODUCED IN THE BODY

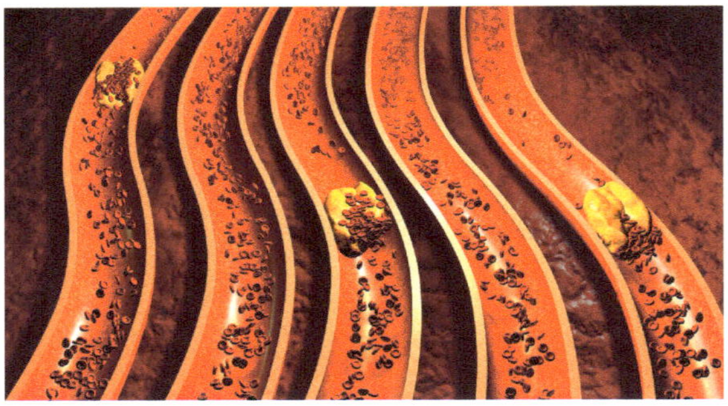

Cholesterol is known to be a yellowish, waxy, fat-like substance made in the liver that our body actually needs to maintain good health. It helps to make the walls of our cells, various tissues in the body, hormones, vitamin D and bile acid. The key is to control how much cholesterol we maintain in our bodies.

When we eat too many fatty foods, don't exercise enough, become overweight and engage in habits like smoking and drinking, we put ourselves at risk for developing high cholesterol. High cholesterol may also be a genetic inheritance, but it can be properly maintained with a healthy lifestyle.

Our liver makes all the cholesterol our bodies need. The two main proteins of cholesterol are low-density lipoproteins (LDL) and high-density lipoproteins (HDL).

WHAT IS MOST IMPORTANT TO YOU IN THIS READING?

MISCONCEPTIONS ABOUT CHOLESTEROL

CHOLESTEROL ISN'T A CONCERN FOR CHILDREN

Inherited cholesterol is called "Familial hypercholesterolemia." According to the American Hearts Association, this is a condition underdiagnosed and undertreated worldwide. Once identified, children with this condition may require aggressive treatment with medications.

WAIT UNTIL MIDDLE AGE TO CHECK CHOLESTEROL

The American Heart Association recommends all adults 20 and older have their cholesterol (and other risk factors) checked every four to six years as long as risks remain low. Work with your doctor to determine your risk for cardiovascular disease and stroke.

ONLY MEN SHOULD WORRY ABOUT CHOLESTEROL

Atherosclerosis typically occurs in women vs men, cardiovascular disease remains the leading cause of death in women. Weight gain also contributes to higher levels. Women nearing menopause should have their cholesterol levels checked more often than those in premenopausal state.

GOOD LDL VS BAD LDL

Low-density lipoprotein (LDL) is referred to as the "bad" cholesterol. However, it serves a purpose in our bodies and only becomes bad when there is too much of it found in our bloodstream.

TRANSPORTS FATS

LDL carries fats that we need through our bloodstream to various cells in the body. Fats can not move on their own.

MORE CHOLESTEROL

LDL particles contain a large amount of cholesterol and a smaller amount of proteins. Fat attracts fat.

HEALTHY LDL LEVEL

Most adults should keep their LDL below 100 milligrams per deciliter (mg/dL). If you have a history of atherosclerosis, your LDL should be below 70 mg/dL.

LDL CHOLESTEROL LEVELS

- Normal: Below 100 mg/dL.
- Near optimal: 100 – 129 mg/dL.
- Borderline high: 130 – 159 mg/dL.
- High: 160 – 189 mg/dL.
- Very high: 190 mg/dL or higher.

VS

TRANSPORTING FATS

Transporting too much fat through our bloodstream can contribute to plaque buildup in our artieries.

TOO MUCH CHOLESTEROL

Too much LDL can clog the arteries increasing the risk of a stroke, heart attack, high blood pressure or heart problems.

UNHEALTHY LDL LEVEL

An LDL level above 100 mg/dL raises your risk of cardiovascular disease.

WHAT YOU EAT

Fatty meats, fried foods, processed foods, pastries, fast food are harmful for your cholesterol levels.

BODY WEIGHT

Being overweight and obese raises your cholesterol levels. Learn the body weight that is proper for your size, gender and age.

READING BLOOD TEST RESULTS LIKE...???

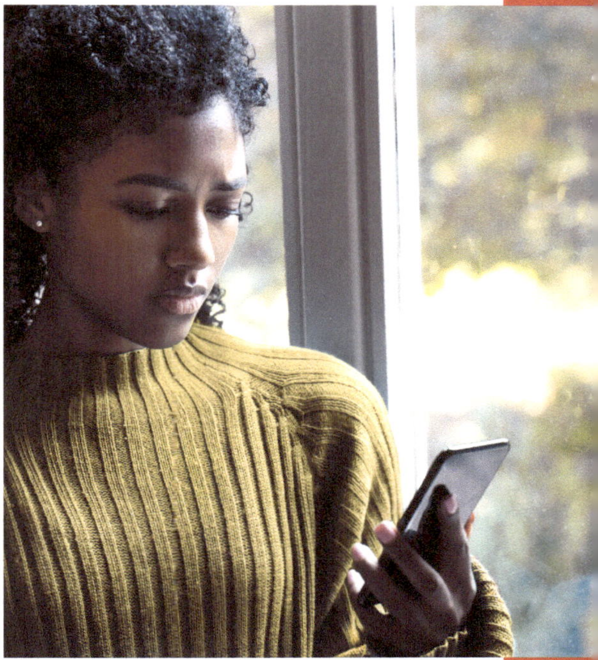

INTERPRETING BLOOD TEST RESULTS

Trying to read and understand blood test results can be stressful. Most times, the test ranges are listed to inform you if you're in a good or not so good range. Doctors should explain your results to you and help you to fix any issues that may be present. Let's take a look at what some tests are testing for.

IRON

You may be familiar with seeing the name ferritin on your blood test for iron. Ferritin looks for iron storage in the body. The CBC test is looking for blood counts to ensure you're not at risk for anemia.

The transferrin test measures the amount of protein transferrin in the blood. This is needed to check if the liver is making transferrin. The liver does so to get more iron into the blood when your iron is running low.

The TIBC initials you may see on your iron test is measuring the bloods ability to attach itself to iron and transport it around the body.

CHOLESTEROL

Cholesterol tests are called lipid profiles. Lipids are cholesterols & triglycerides better known as fats and oils. These things become dangerous when they begin to build up in the blood. The lipid profile test is looking for how much fat is in the blood to help evaluate cardiovascular health.

LOWER YOUR CHOLESTEROL QUICKLY WITH SOLUBLE FIBER

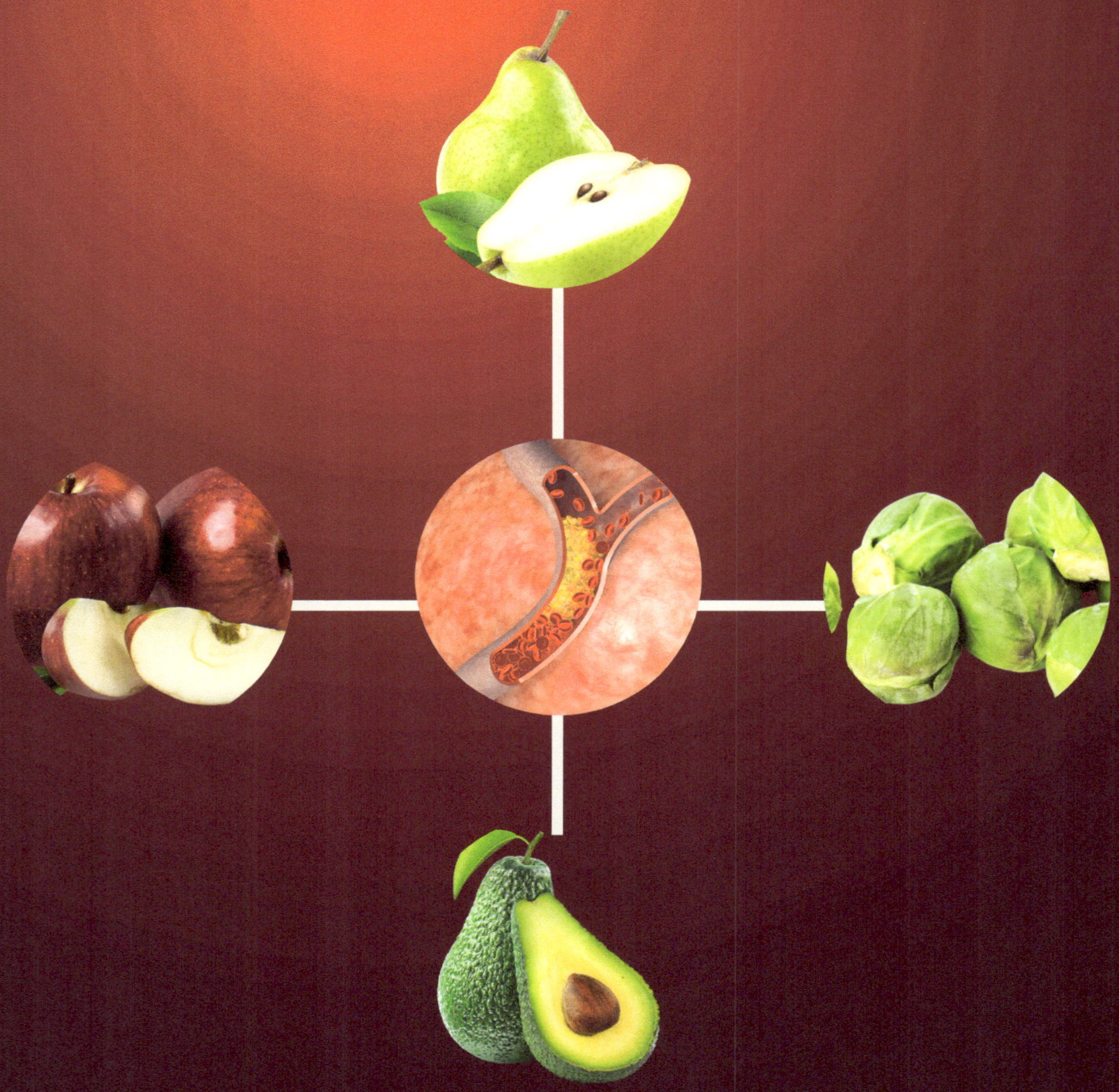

THREE HERBS THAT LOWER CHOLESTEROL

01

Ginseng

Mixed with other herbs, ginseng has been used in Asian medicine for centuries. Studies have proven that ginseng supports healthy levels of LDL cholesterol and HDL cholesterol. It is also known to help with heart health and diabetes.

02

Hawthorn

This is a plant that can be used in its entirety, both the berries and the leaves. Its berries antioxidant properties helps with the cardiovascular system and the entire plant supports healthy levels of total cholesterol, LDL cholesterol and triglycerides which are the fats in the blood.

03

Ginger

Ginger is a SUPER herb with so many medicinal purposes. As it relates to cholesterol it helps to reduce the high levels of LDL and boost the levels of HDL. You can take ginger raw, as a powder, tea, tincture or supplement.

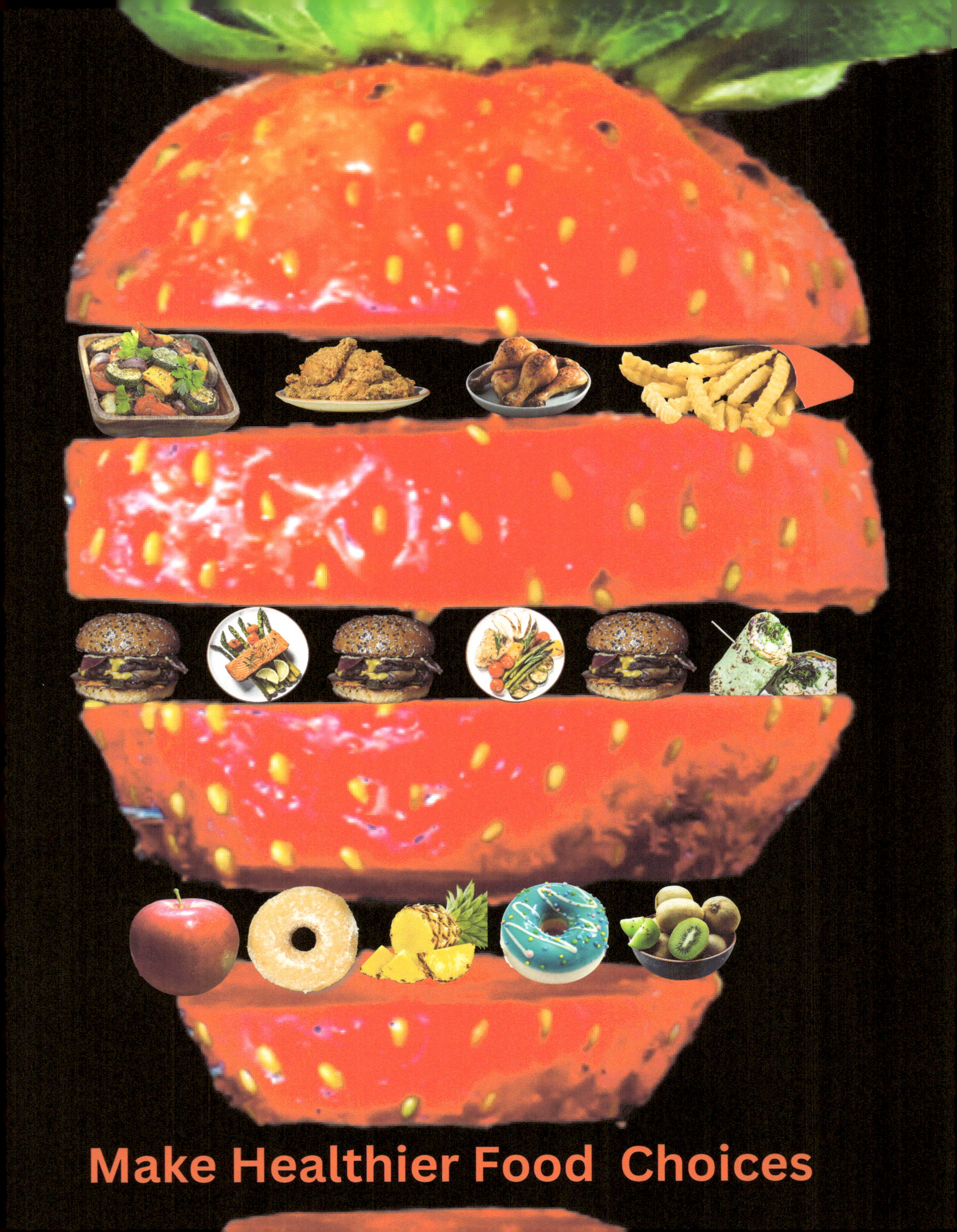
Make Healthier Food Choices

CHOOSE WHAT MAINTAINS HEALTHY CHOLESTEROL LEVELS

ENJOY!

SUGGESTED DISH OPTIONS

Eating healthy is always the goal. Knowing what you eat and the purpose it serves in your body is always a plus. Here are some healthy meal choices to help you along your journey!

SAUTEED BROCCOLI

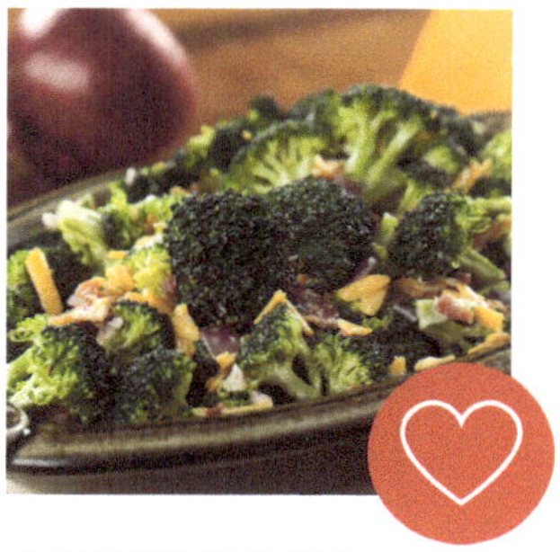

INGREDIENTS

- 2 tablespoons olive oil
- 6 cups broccoli florets
- 1 teaspoons sea salt or to taste
- 3 garlic cloves minced
- 1 teaspoon black pepper to taste
- 1 to 2 tablespoons freshly squeezed lemon juice

DIRECTIONS

- Heat a large skillet over low-medium heat. Add the olive oil and garlic.
- Add broccoli after cooking garlic for 1-2 min on a low fire.
- Sprinkle with salt and pepper, and allow the broccoli to cook on medium fire.
- Add lemon juice once broccoli is half way done.
- Cook until broccoli is done. (pierce with a fork) *Don't allow broccoli to get mushy.

FRUIT SALAD

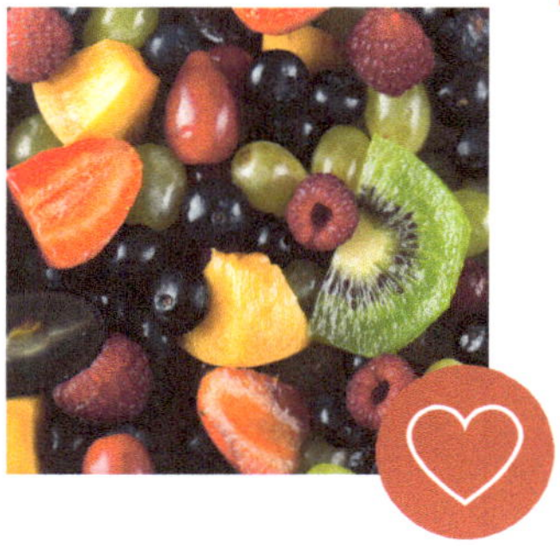

INGRIDIENTS

- fresh strawberries
- fresh pineapple
- fresh blueberries
- red grapes
- kiwis
- mandarin oranges

DIRECTIONS

- Add all fruit to a large mixing bowl.
- In a small mixing bowl, whisk together the honey, lime zest and lime juice.
- Pour over fruit and toss to evenly coat, serve immediately.

FRUIT SALAD LIME SAUCE

INGRIDIENTS

- 1/4 cup honey
- 2 tsp lime zest (zest of 2 medium limes)
- 2 Tbsp fresh lime juice

DIRECTIONS

- Combine all ingredients in a bowl and whisk together.

!

Stay committed! You can do this! You deserve to live a healthier lifestyle!

CHOOSE WHAT MAINTAINS HEALTHY CHOLESTEROL LEVELS

AVOCADO TOAST

INGRIDIENTS

- 2 Whole wheat bread slices
- 1 Ripe Avocado
- ½ teaspoon Garlic powder
- 2 teaspoon Lemon or Lime juice
- ⅛ teaspoon Sea Salt to taste
- 2 tablespoon Red onion finely chopped
- ¼ teaspoon Red pepper flakes to taste
- ½ tablespoon Cilantro
- ½ teaspoon Olive oil apply after toasting the bread slices

DIRECTIONS

- Remove the pit from 1 ripe avocado. Using a spoon, scoop out the flesh, add it to a bowl, and using a fork, mash it till it's smooth as you like.
- Add lemon juice, garlic powder, and salt to taste and mix well.
- Add ½ teaspoon Garlic powder, 2 teaspoon Lemon or Lime juice, ⅛ teaspoon Sea Salt
- Toast the bread until crisp and golden brown in a toaster, or toast in a pan on medium heat with olive oil.
- Spread the mashed avocado on top of the toast. Garnish it with red onions, cilantro, and red pepper flakes, or use any other topping ideas mentioned in the post.
- 2 tablespoon Red onion, ½ tablespoon Cilantro or coriander leaves, ¼ teaspoon Red pepper flakes

Unhealthy Eating Tracker

Food Item	s	m	t	w	t	f	s

Wellness Questions

to Ask Yourself

- Who inspires me the most?
- What am I grateful for today?
- What am I most committed to?
- What do I like most about myself?
- What will I do today to bring myself joy?

SELF-CARE PLANNER

DATE: ______________________ S M T W T F S

THINGS THAT MADE ME HAPPY TODAY

- ______________________
- ______________________
- ______________________

WATER INTAKE

1L 2L 3L

TODAY'S MOOD

SELF-CARE ACTIVITIES

- ______________________
- ______________________
- ______________________
- ______________________

DAILY NUTRITION

Vegetables ______________________

Fruit ______________________

Protein ______________________

Fluids ______________________

HABITS TO START

- ______________________
- ______________________
- ______________________
- ______________________

HABITS TO STOP

- ______________________
- ______________________
- ______________________
- ______________________

Daily Journal

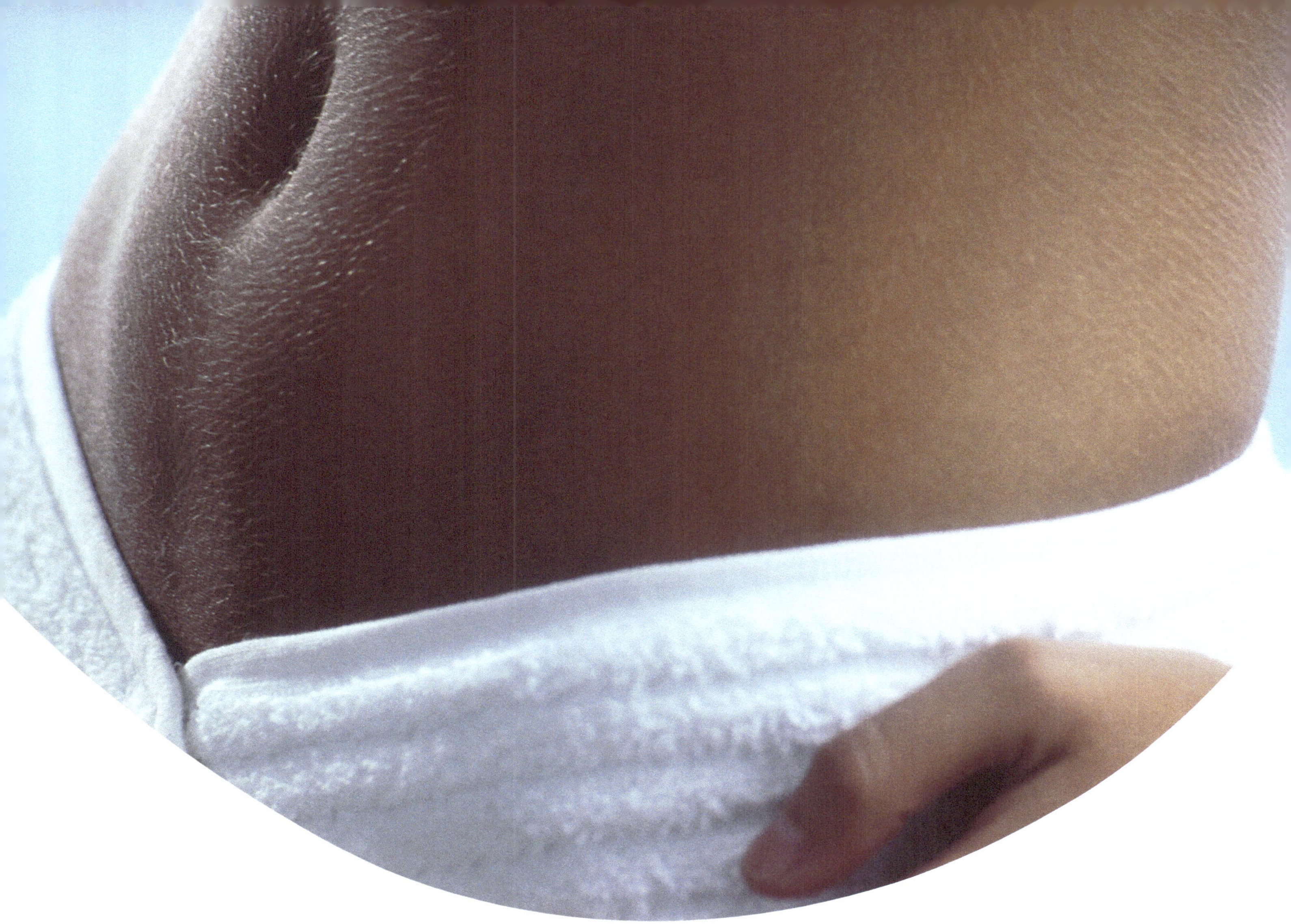

WOMB HEALTH

The uterus is where the woman becomes a co-creator with God.
Embrace it, nurture it and fall in love with your gift to this world.

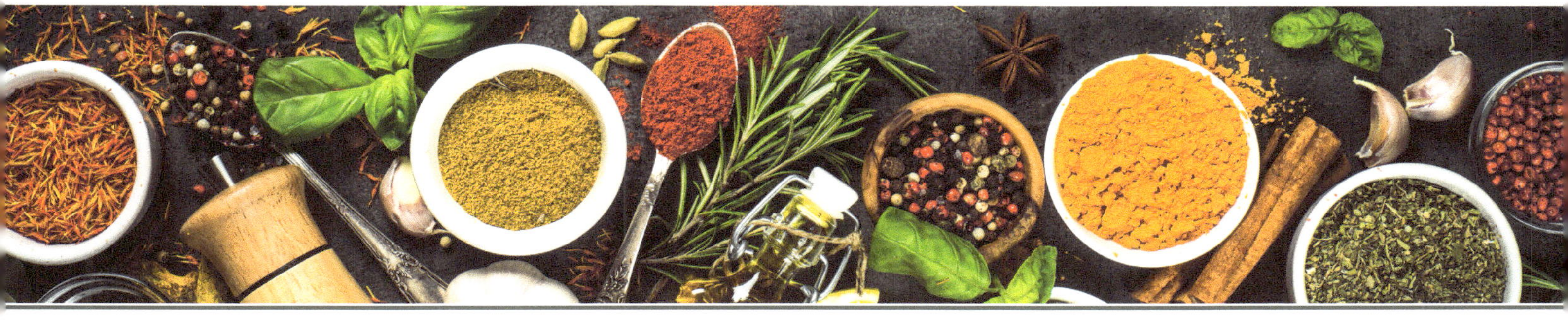

SPECIAL NOTE ABOUT YOUR WOMB

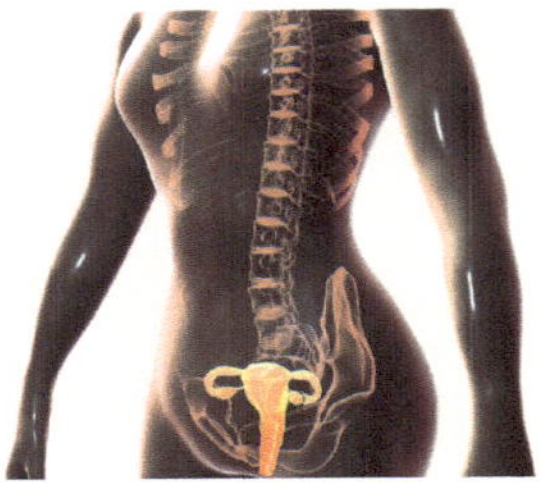

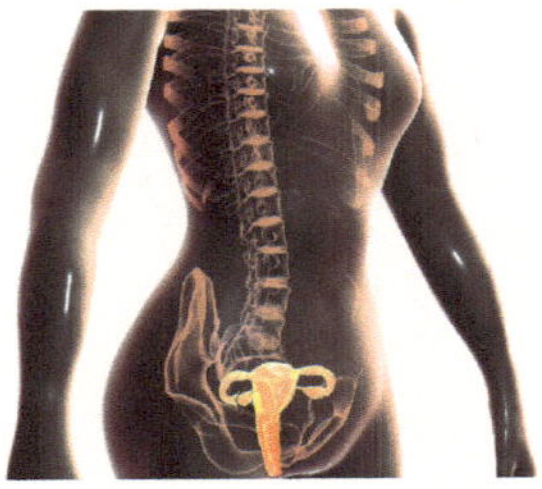

The female reproductive system is made up of a number of different parts, most notably the vagina, uterus and egg producing ovaries. Your reproductive system contains the largest and smallest human cells in the body. Your vagina is highly acidic. Its pH averages between 3.8 & 4.5. Anything that changes your vagina's pH balance can throw off bacteria levels and lead to infection. Actions such as douching, using scented products and deodorants around the vagina, wearing tight non-breathable clothing, or using irritating products can all contribute to pH imbalance.

When we eat the wrong foods, carry negative thoughts, have multiple sex partners and unprotected sex, we damage one of the most important systems of the body. Our reproductive system has the responsibility of bringing new life into this world and we should protected it as much as possible. Once a woman is passed child birthing years, you still want to continue to take care of your system. You don't want to develop weak bones, urinary tract infections or cancers.

WHAT DID YOU LEARN FROM THIS READING & WHAT WAS MOST IMPORTANT TO YOU?

CHECKLIST TO KEEP A HEALTHY REPRODUCTIVE SYSTEM

Favorable reproductive health means that your reproductive system is not only, more than free from disease but functioning well.

MANAGE STRESS LEVELS

Stress alters your normal menstrual cycle and causes hormonal imbalances.

GO FOR REGULAR SCREENINGS

This can ensure early detection of any condition, which gives you a better chance of survival.

INCREASE CALCIUM & MAGNESIUM

It is essential that these two vital minerals are combined, magnesium provides the mechanism that enables the control or moderation of calcium levels in the cells.

STOP SMOKING & DRINKING ALCOHOL

Smoking and alcohol consumption is linked to many reproductive health issues.

MAINTAIN A HEALTHY DIET

WHAT YOU EAT MATTERS! EAT MORE FIBER RICH FOODS & REDUCE PROCESSED FOOD INTAKE.

NOTES TO SELF

QUESTIONS TO ASK YOUR OBGYN IF YOU HAVE ENDOMETRIOSIS

1 WHAT'S CAUSING MY SYMPTOMS?

This is an important question to ask, because endometriosis is sometimes mistaken for other conditions like pelvic inflammatory disease or ovarian cysts. You may also want to avoid what may be causing your symptoms, to prevent yourself from having them. Always seek a second medical opinion.

2 WHAT CAN THE TREATMENT OPTIONS DO FOR ME?

Everyone is different. Do not allow a doctor to treat you like you belong to a particular group of people. Ask to be cared for like the unique individual you are. The primary goal of treatment for endometriosis is to stop the growth and activity of the lesions.

3 WHAT LIFESTYLE CHANGES MIGHT HELP?

The ultimate goal is to get better and become free from disease. You don't want to engage in activity that will make your condition worse.

4 WHAT AM I TO DO IF MY SYMPTOMS DO NOT IMPROVE?

You want to let your doctor know if your symptoms do not go away or if they worsen. Herbs like chamomile, peppermint and ashwagandha are known for helping to relieve the pain associated with endometriosis.

5 WILL THIS AFFECT MY FERTILITY? IF SO, HOW WILL WE TREAT THAT?

Women with endometriosis are known to be able to have children, even though this may be a difficult task. Endometriosis can damage the egg or sperm. Or it can cause inflammation which interferes with the delicate balance of hormones that women need to become pregnant.

There are medications, herbs & lifestyle changes that can treat fertility issues caused by endometriosis.

SOME FOODS THAT FEED FIBROIDS

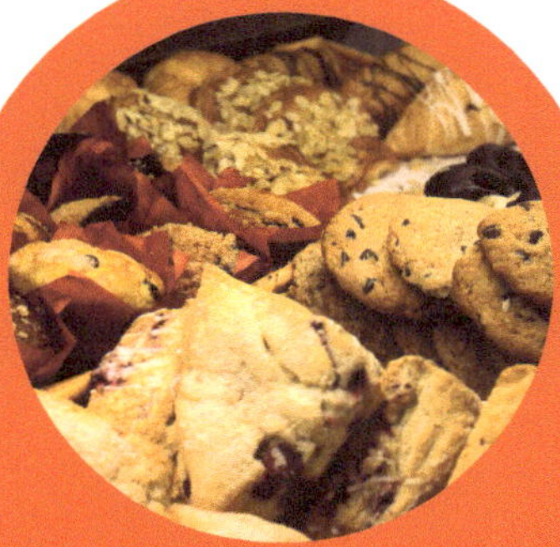

REFINED CARBO-HYDRATES

The types of foods that fall into this category are white sugars, white bread, cakes, cookies, etc. These types of foods alter your estrogen levels causing the fibroids to increase in size. This list also includes potato chips and anything that has corn syrup in it. These foods create a candy store in your blood stream for fibroids to feed on.

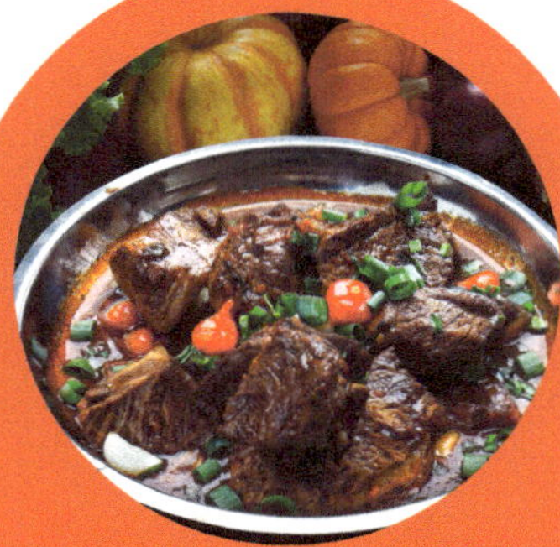

RED MEATS

Red meat is known to have added hormones to it, particularly estrogen. It contains high levels of estrogen. The high fat content generally found in these meats create inflammation in the body, which can worsen the symptoms that accompany fibroids. You may want to focus on avoiding the types of foods that spike hormone levels.

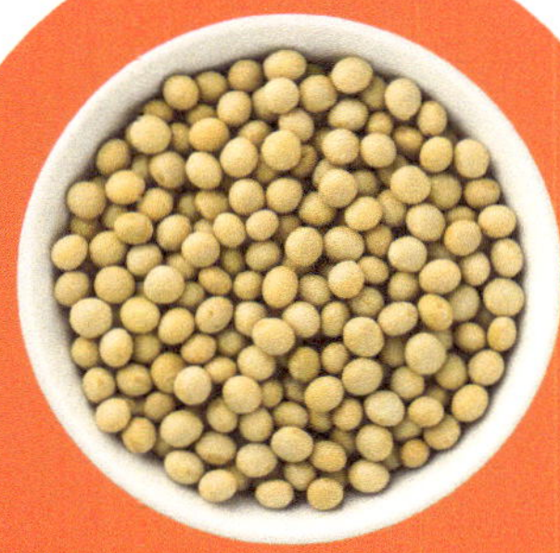

SOY

Soy has phytoestrogens in it. These compounds act like estrogen in your body. High estrogen levels boost fibroid growth. Estrogen's job is to stimulate development in the uterine lining during your menstrual cycle. New studies show soy can cause infertility, trigger early puberty, and impact fetal development.

!

So far, there is no absolute way to prevent fibroids from developing. However, having a healthy diet and lifestyle can definitely help. Vitamin D deficiencies also increases the risks of developing fibroids. Other foods that are considered to worsen fibroids are foods high in salt, foods containing Monosodium Glutamate (MSG), caffeine, alcohol and high fat dairy products.

HEALTHY FOODS FOR FIBROIDS

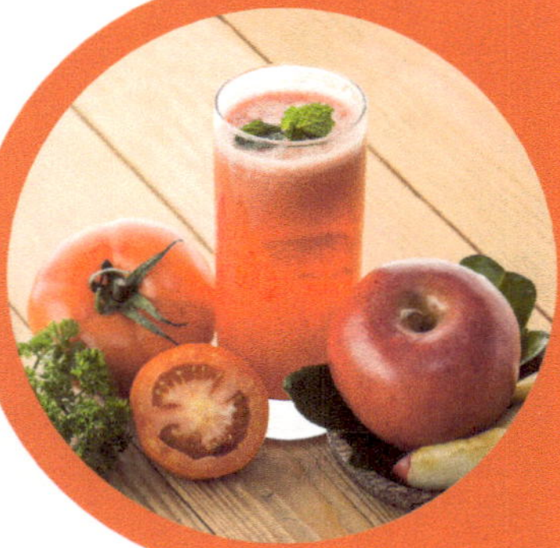

FRUITS & VEGETABLES

Eating plenty of fruits like apples and tomatoes and or cruciferous vegetables like broccoli and cabbage, could lower the risk of developing fibroids. These types of fruits and vegetables may also improve your symptoms. Make your food choices organic!

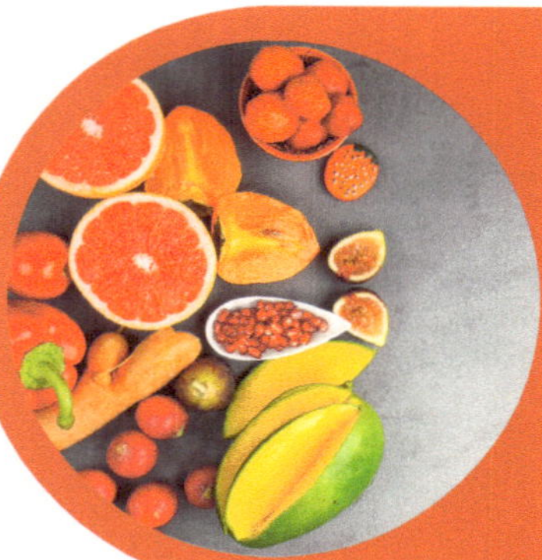

HIGH FIBER

Fiber may help prevent and slow down the growth of fibroids. Fiber can help you get rid of excess estrogen in the body through your stool. It binds to the estrogen and stops your small intestines from reabsorbing the estrogen into your blood stream. High fiber diets also promote weightloss. Being overweight is also linked to fibroids.

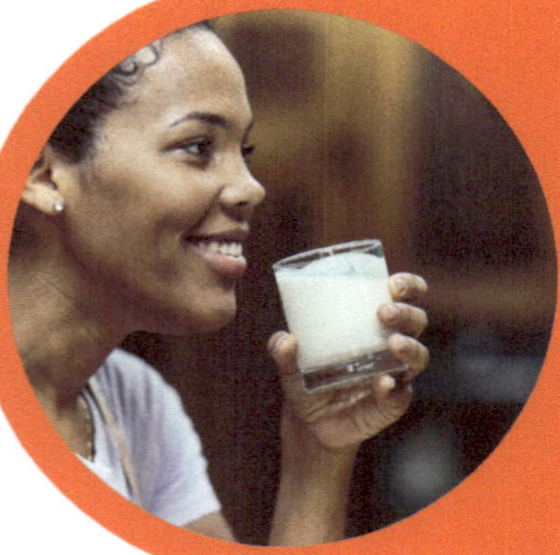

VITAMIN D

Low vitamin D levels puts us at risk for fibroids. Recent studies show that vitamin D supplementation shrinks fibroids and prevents them from becoming more severe. Make note that there's no meaningful difference between vitamin D3 and just vitamin D.

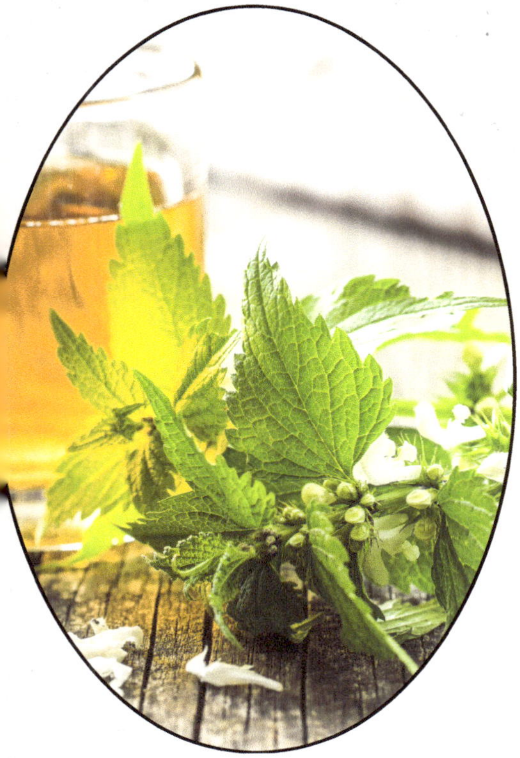

1. Nettle

Known to be one of natures greatest multivitamins. It's high in iron and good for fertility and postpartum. It is also known to be good for kidney health. This herb can be taken as a tea, tincture, powder extract or even a seasoning on food. It is advised to avoid eating this herb's fresh leaves because it may cause irritation to the digestive tract.

2. Red Raspberry Leaf

This plant is power packed with vitamin C, quercetin, ellagic acid, magnesium, potassium, vitamin K, calcium and iron. It helps with PMS, premenstrual bloating, heavy period flows, endometriosis and cardiovascular disorders. You can receive the best results from this herb when used as fresh leaves or fresh dried. You can chop it up and put in on top of a salad or other types of foods. You can also drink it as a tea or tincture.

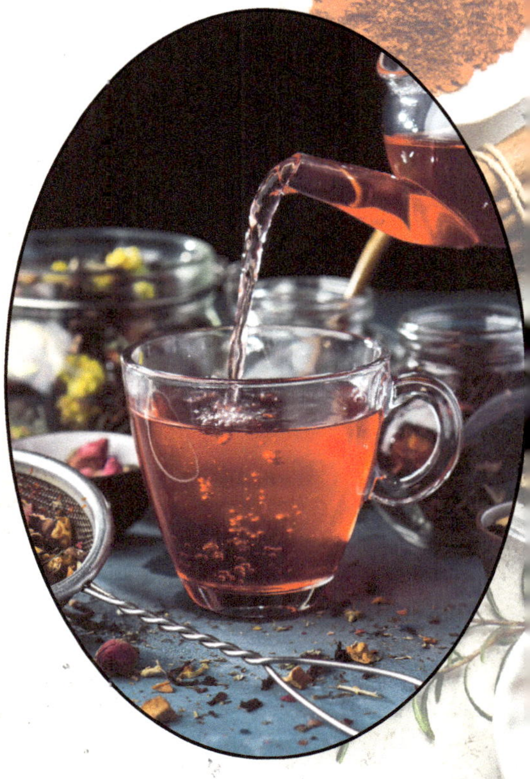

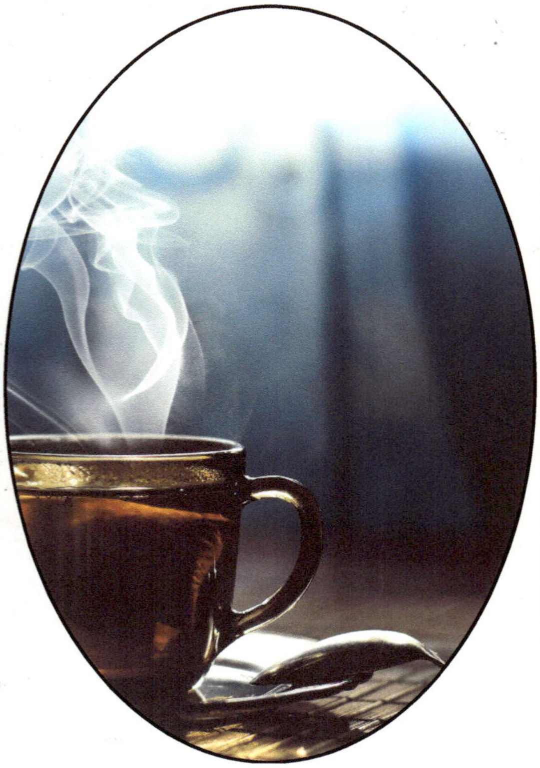

3. Shatavari

This herb, native to India, is good for women in all stages of life. It's amazing for womb health. This amazing herb curbs physical and psychological stress which is often associated with hormonal imbalances. Shatavari helps to balance sluggish or heavy menstrual flows. It improves reproductive health, helps with PCOS, follicular growth & development, infertility, vaginal dryness and hotflashes.

4. Black Cohosh

This botanical plant is used by the Native Americans. It can be used as a hormone replacement therapy to support menopause. It can help with PMS, PCOS and painful menstruation. It also helps with colds, rheumatism, kidney disorders, menstrual disorders, lactation, hot flashes, sleep disorders, body pains, irritability and mood swings. Can be taken as a tea, tincture or capsule.

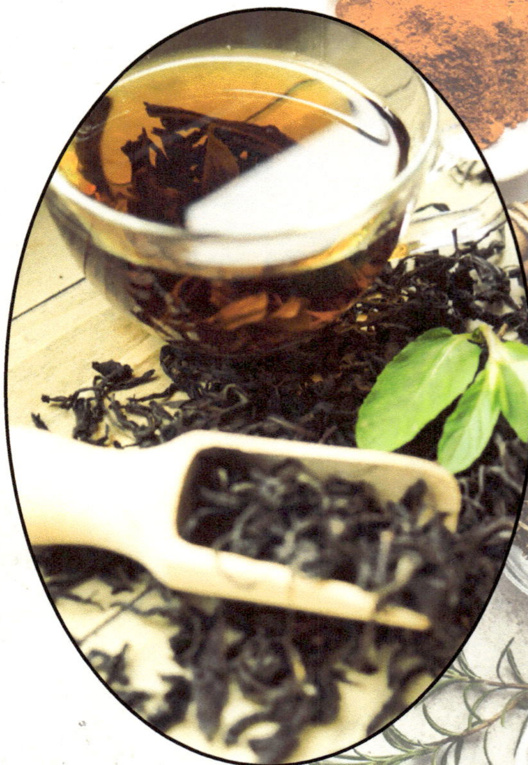

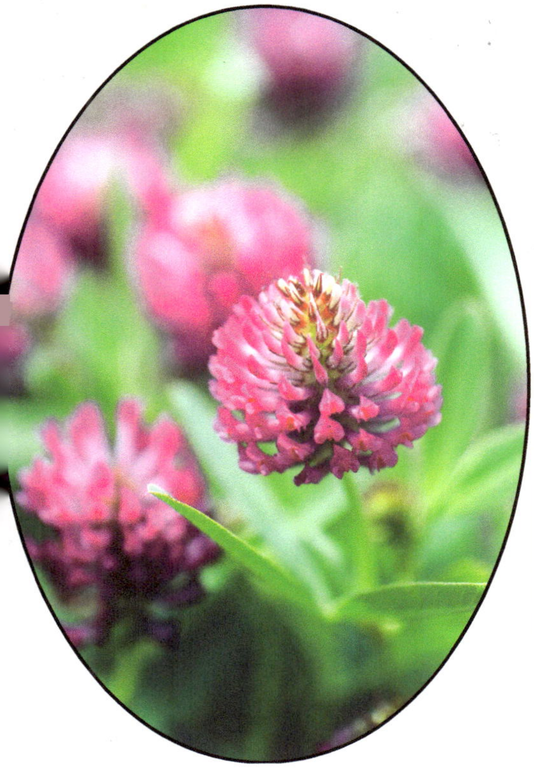

5. Red Clover

This herb is an excellent multi-vitamin. It contains good levels of calcium, vitamin C, beta-carotene, a whole spectrum of B vitamins, and trace minerals such as magnesium, zinc, copper, selenium & magnesium. Red clover may help with hot flashes, mood swings & night sweats. It can be used as a tonic to prepare the uterus for pregnancy. This herb is best taken as a tea of fresh herb tincture.

6. Vitex (Chasteberry)

This berry is dynamic for women's health. It's also known to boost memory, learning & cognition. Vitex directly enhances the primary gland that regulates hormone secretion, which is the pituitary gland. It can be used ONLY in the first trimester of pregnancy to help prevent miscarriages. After the first trimester it should not be taken. It stimulates lactation, can help bring back menstruation from amenorrhea, may help with PMS, PCOS, fertility challenges, irregular menstrual cycles & menopause symptoms. Best taken as a tincture or capsule.

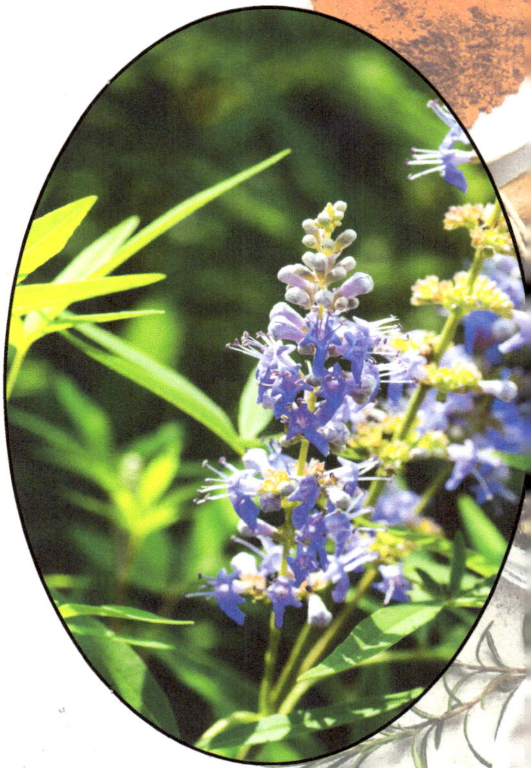

7. Cramp Bark (V. Opulus)

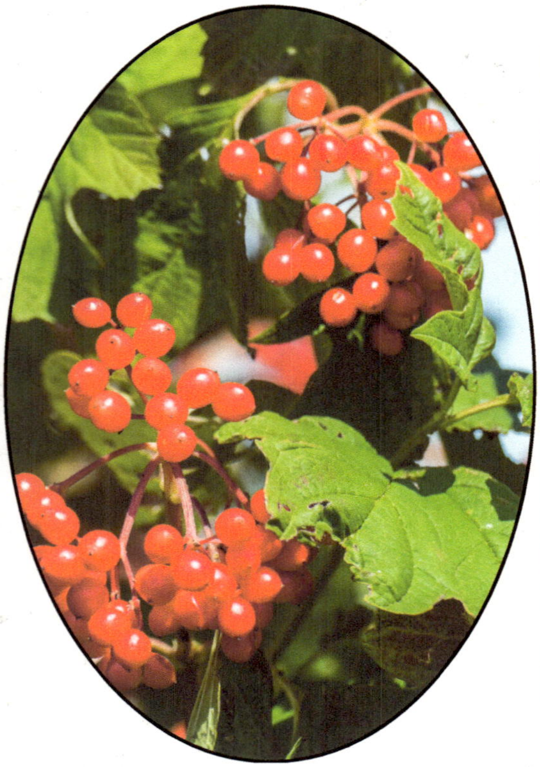

This wonderful herb is used to ease cramps and discomfort throughout the body. It is also known to be good for the health of lymph glands. Cramp bark has the ability to ease discomforts associated with menstrual cramps. It is excellent at toning the muscles of the uterus and easing spasms all over the body, working as a muscle relaxer. This herb has been useful in easing digestive complaints, promoting respiratory & heart health & urinary tract health. Jojoba oil infused with this herb can be good for topical use for muscle discomfort. This herb is best taken as a tea or tincture.

Quick Recipe

- Simmer 1/2 cup of cramp bark in 2 cups of water in a covered pan for 20 minutes.
- Strain the bark and allow to cool slightly.
- Soak a cloth in the tea and apply to the affected area for at least 20 - 30 minutes.
- Place a warm towel or heating pad over the cloth to keep it warm longer.

9 TIPS FOR WOMB HEALTH

TIP 1

OMEGA 3- FATTY ACIDS

INCREASES BLOOD FLOW TO THE UTERUS. PREVENTS MENSTRUAL PAIN. REDUCES INFLAMMATION

TIP 2

AVOID XENOESTROGENS

THEY INTERRUPT OUR HORMONE BALANCE, CREATING FIBROIDS & HEAVY FLOWS

TIP 3

AVOID BIRTH CONTROL PILLS

CAN INTERRUPT THE BODY'S NATURAL HORMONE BALANCE AND INCREASE THE CHANCES OF DEVELOPING FIBROIDS

TIP 4

DON'T STRESS YOUR BLADDER

A FULL BLADDER CAN PLACE PRESSURE ON THE UTERUS AND CAUSE THE UTERUS TO SHIFT OUT OF POSITION, IF URINE IS HELD TOO LONG

TIP 5

DO NOT SIT TOO LONG

SITTING TOO LONG PREVENTS BLOOD FLOWING TO THE PELVIC, INCREASING THE CHANCES OF ENDOMETRIOSIS

TIP 6

WARM YOUR UTERUS

COLD TO/IN THE UTERUS CAN LEAD TO PAINFUL PERIODS AND INFERTILITY. IT ALSO PREVENTS BLOODFLOW

TIP 7

BUILD UTERUS IMMUNITY

VITAMIN C
VITAMIN D
AVOCADOS
BERRIES
APPLES
IRON
B12

TIP 8

EXERCISE THE PELVIC FLOOR

YOGA
KEGEL EXERCISE
WALL SQUATS
IT'S VERY IMPORTANT TO MAINTAIN A HEALTHY WEIGHT

TIP 9

ONE CLEAN SEXUAL PARTNER

THE FOLDS OF A MAN'S PENIS CARRIES BACTERIA IF NOT CLEANED CORRECTLY. HE SHOULD WASH BEFORE SEX

MY WOMB HEALTH GOAL IS

WHY IS THIS GOAL IMPORTANT?

STEPS TO TAKE

- [ ]
- [ ]
- [ ]
- [ ]
- [ ]

CHALLENGES	RESPONSES

DEADLINE ____________ MARK AS COMPLETE ☐

Self Love Questions

In what ways do I show love for myself?

Do I feel guilty if I put my needs first?

How important is my own happiness?

When was the last time I gave a compliment to myself?

Self Love Journey

I feel loved when...

I feel blessed when...

I feel confident when...

I feel proud when...

I feel safe when...

Self Love Checklist

Activity	S	M	T	W	T	F	S
Alone time	☐	☐	☐	☐	☐	☐	☐
Declutter	☐	☐	☐	☐	☐	☐	☐
Dine out	☐	☐	☐	☐	☐	☐	☐
Exercise	☐	☐	☐	☐	☐	☐	☐
Make art	☐	☐	☐	☐	☐	☐	☐
Meditation	☐	☐	☐	☐	☐	☐	☐
Read books	☐	☐	☐	☐	☐	☐	☐
Sleep in	☐	☐	☐	☐	☐	☐	☐

Notes

FUN & ROMANTIC

LOVE QUESTIONS CARD GAME

27 UNIQUE CARDS

LOVE QUESTIONS

WHAT MAKES YOU FEEL MOST LOVED?

LOVE QUESTIONS

WHEN DID YOU KNOW YOU LOVED YOURSELF?

BE SINCERE & HAVE FUN

LOVE QUESTIONS

IS THERE A SMELL THAT INSTANTLY RELAXES YOU?

LOVE QUESTIONS

WHEN WAS THE LAST

LOVE QUESTIONS

WHAT'S YOUR

LOVE QUESTIONS

WHEN WAS THE FIRST

LOVE QUESTIONS

WHAT MAKES YOU FEEL MOST LOVED?

BE SINCERE & HAVE FUN

LOVE QUESTIONS

WHEN DID YOU KNOW YOU LOVED YOURSELF?

BE SINCERE & HAVE FUN

LOVE QUESTIONS

IS THERE A SMELL THAT INSTANTLY RELAXES YOU?

BE SINCERE & HAVE FUN

LOVE QUESTIONS

WHEN WAS THE LAST TIME YOU CRIED?

BE SINCERE & HAVE FUN

LOVE QUESTIONS

WHAT'S YOUR LANGUAGE OF LOVE?

BE SINCERE & HAVE FUN

LOVE QUESTIONS

WHEN WAS THE FIRST TIME YOU FELL IN LOVE?

BE SINCERE & HAVE FUN

LOVE QUESTIONS

WHAT IS YOUR FAVORITE THING ABOUT YOURSELF?

BE SINCERE & HAVE FUN

LOVE QUESTIONS

WHAT WAS YOUR BEST BIRTHDAY?

BE SINCERE & HAVE FUN

LOVE QUESTIONS

WHAT DO YOU LOOK FOR WITHIN YOURSELF?

BE SINCERE & HAVE FUN

LOVE QUESTIONS

DO YOU TRUST YOURSELF?

BE SINCERE & HAVE FUN

LOVE QUESTIONS

WHERE IN THE WORLD DO YOU DESERVE TO TRAVEL?

BE SINCERE & HAVE FUN

LOVE QUESTIONS

WHAT THINGS DO YOU LOOK FORWARD TO EACH DAY?

BE SINCERE & HAVE FUN

LOVE QUESTIONS

WHAT IS YOUR FAVORITE CHILDHOOD MEMORY?

BE SINCERE & HAVE FUN

LOVE QUESTIONS

ARE YOU SATISFIED WITH YOUR OWN INTIMACY?

BE SINCERE & HAVE FUN

LOVE QUESTIONS

WHAT IS YOUR IDEA OF A HEALTHY RELATIONSHIP WITH SELF?

BE SINCERE & HAVE FUN

LOVE QUESTIONS

WHAT SONG DO YOU THINK OF WHEN YOU THINK OF YOURSELF?

BE SINCERE & HAVE FUN

LOVE QUESTIONS

WHAT IS YOUR FAVORITE DATE TIME WITH YOURSELF?

BE SINCERE & HAVE FUN

LOVE QUESTIONS

WHERE IS A PLACE YOU'VE ALWAYS WANTED TO TRAVEL?

BE SINCERE & HAVE FUN

LOVE QUESTIONS

✷

DO YOU CONSIDER "YOU" YOUR BEST FRIEND?

✷

BE SINCERE & HAVE FUN

LOVE QUESTIONS

✷

WHAT IS YOUR DEAREST MEMORY ABOUT YOU AND GOD?

BE SINCERE & HAVE FUN

LOVE QUESTIONS

✷

DO YOU HAVE ANY REGRETS?

✷

BE SINCERE & HAVE FUN

LOVE QUESTIONS

✷

WHAT RELIGIOUS WOMAN REMINDS YOU OF YOURSELF?

BE SINCERE & HAVE FUN

LOVE QUESTIONS

✷

DO YOU THINK YOUR SELF-LOVE HAS GROWN OVER THE YEARS?

BE SINCERE & HAVE FUN

LOVE QUESTIONS

✷

DO YOU HAVE A DREAM THAT YOU NEED HELP WITH?

✷

BE SINCERE & HAVE FUN

LOVE QUESTIONS

✷

WHO ARE YOUR CLOSEST FRIENDS?

✷

BE SINCERE & HAVE FUN

LOVE QUESTIONS

✷

DO YOU BELIEVE IN YOURSELF?

✷

BE SINCERE & HAVE FUN

LOVE QUESTIONS

✷

DO YOU MAKE YOURSELF FEEL SAFE AND PROTECTED?

BE SINCERE & HAVE FUN

Monthly Focus

What is my priority for this month?

How can I improve my confidence?

Reminder:

Resolution:

How can I love myself more?

Things I should keep on doing:

Things I should stop doing:

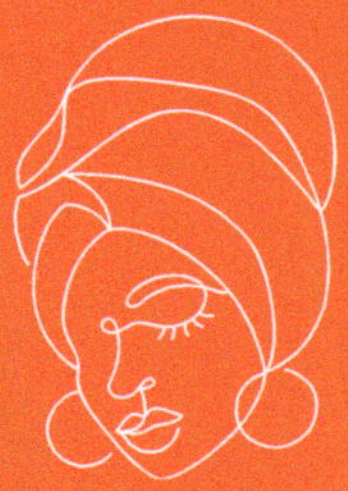

Create A New You

Use the womb of your mind and give birth to a better you!

1 How old is she?

2 Does she have a big or a small family?

3 What music does she like?

4 Where does she live?

5 What is her favorite relax time?

6 What does she do with herself to bring joy?

7 What makes her curious?

8 What is she afraid of?

9 Does she have a superpower? What is it?

10 Is she allergic to something?

11 What does she do when she is bored?

12 What is her favorite food?

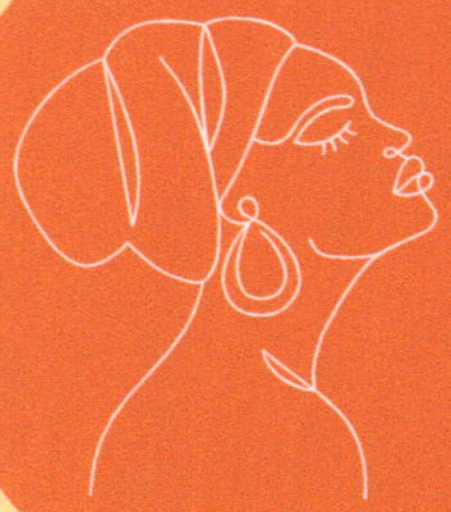

Create a Character

Part 2: Draw your character and describe it using the information from the previous questions.

Describe what you drew.

6 WAYS TO KEEP YOUR BONES Strong & Healthy

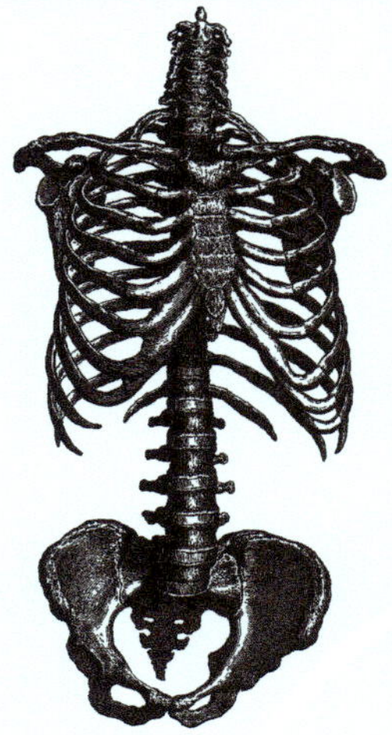

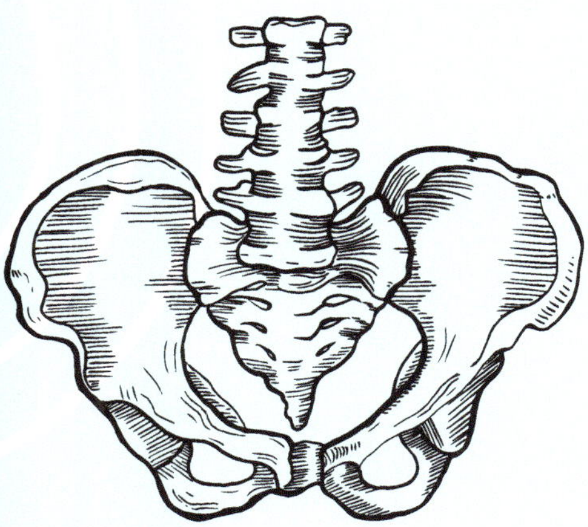

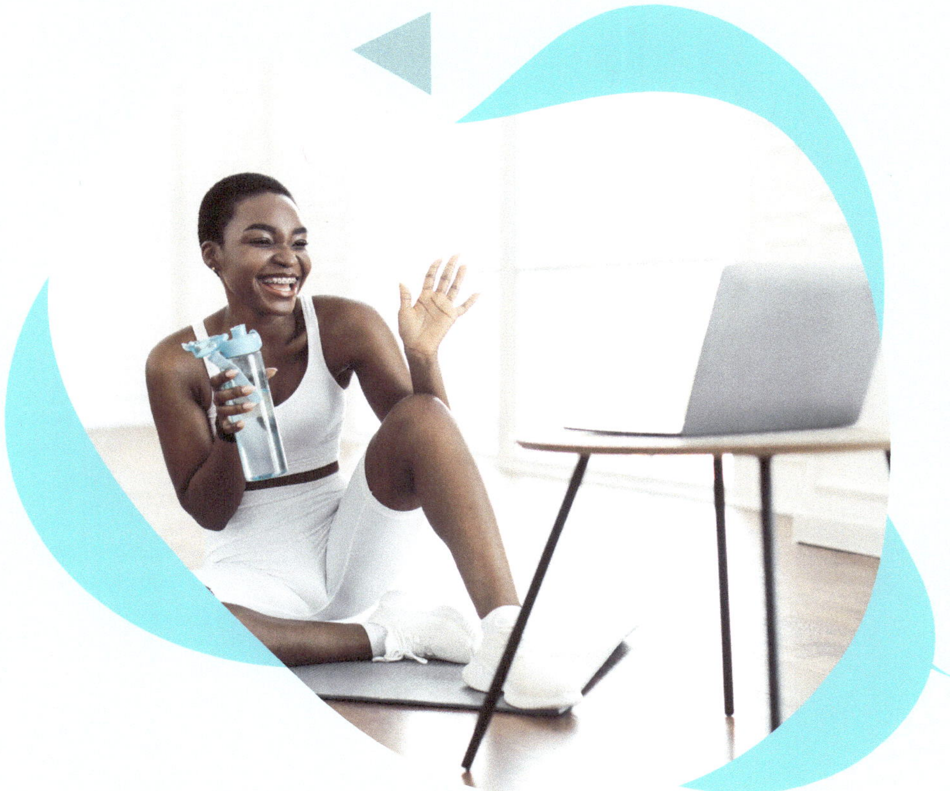

1

Choose calcium-rich

FOOD

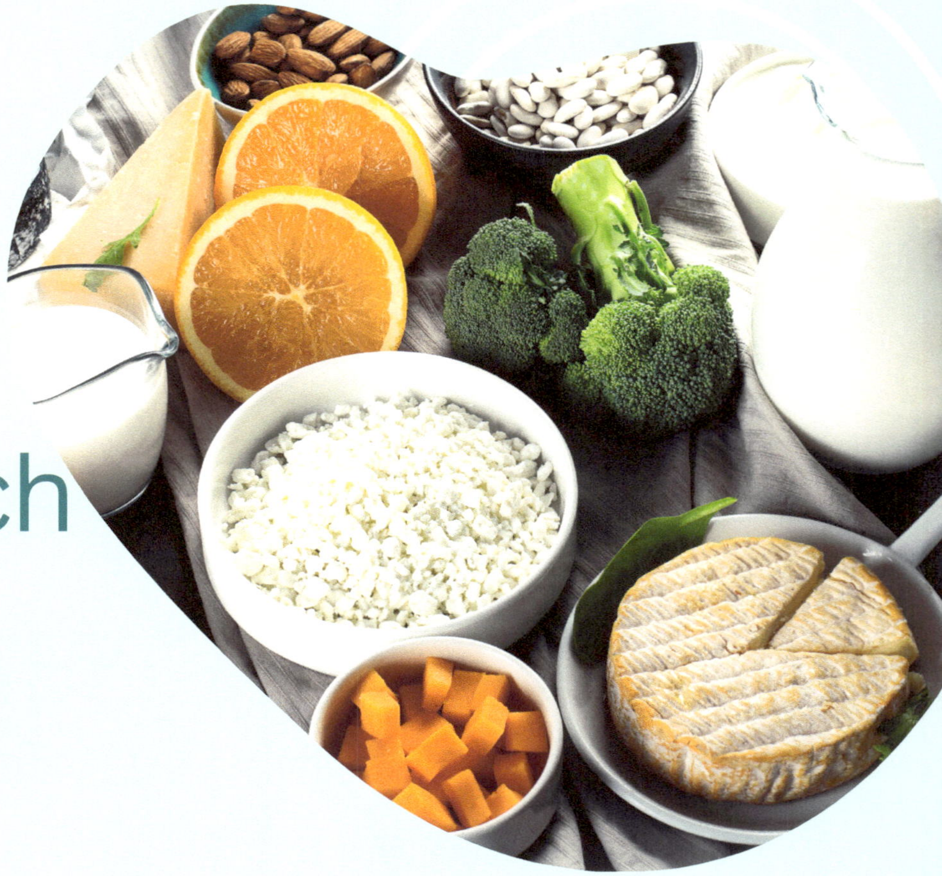

Calcium is the building-block of bones. You can find calcium in foods like:

- Milk
- Yogurt
- Cheese
- Probiotic Kayley
- Winter Squash
- Healthy Smoothies
- Ice Cream (on a treat day)

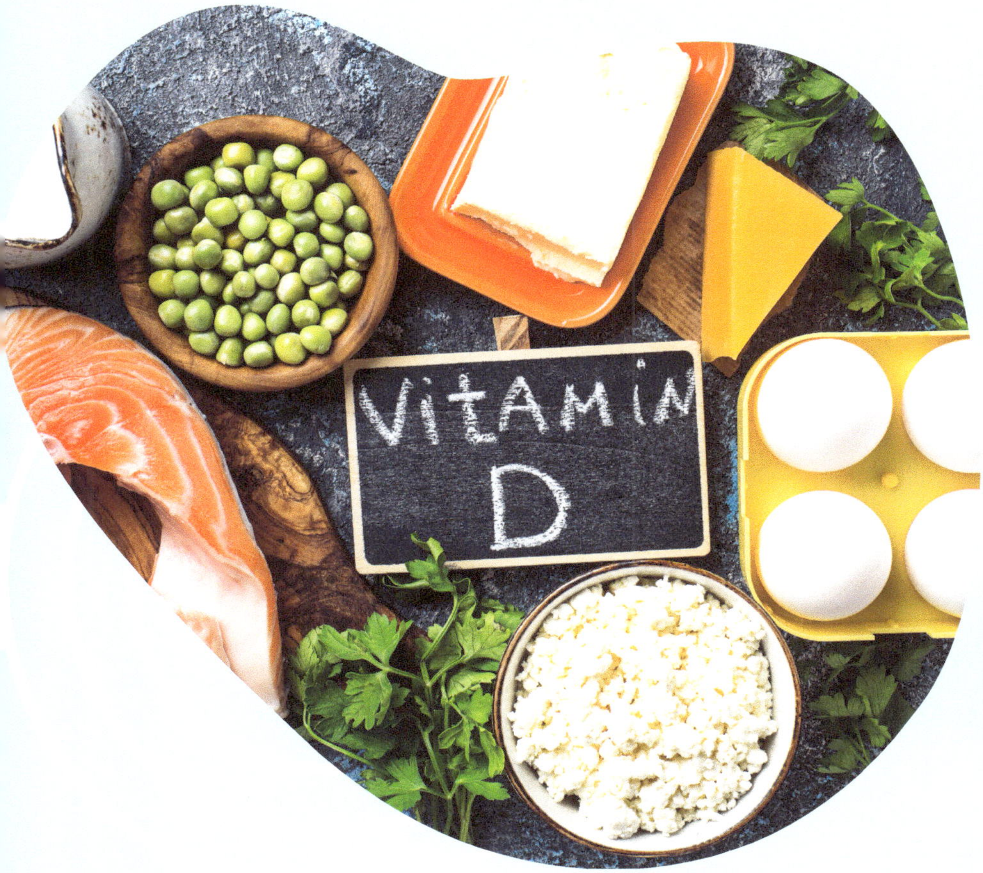

2

Get enough VIT D

Some people have trouble getting enough vitamin D. Health Canada recommends that all adults over the age of 50 take a supplement with 400 IU of vitamin D each day. Speak to a dietitian or health care provider if you do not drink milk or fortified plant-based beverages.

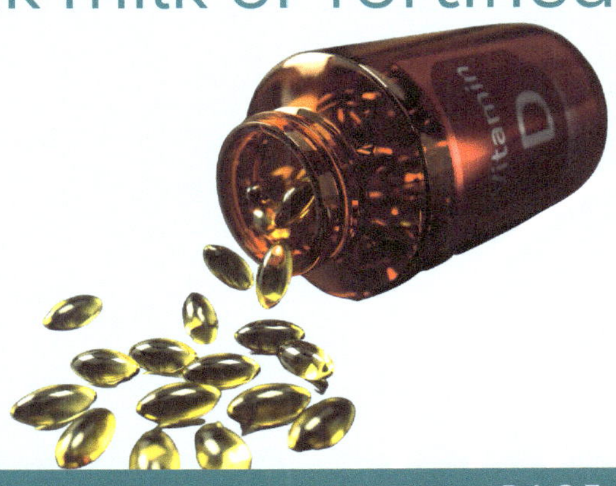

3 Get enough NUTRIENTS

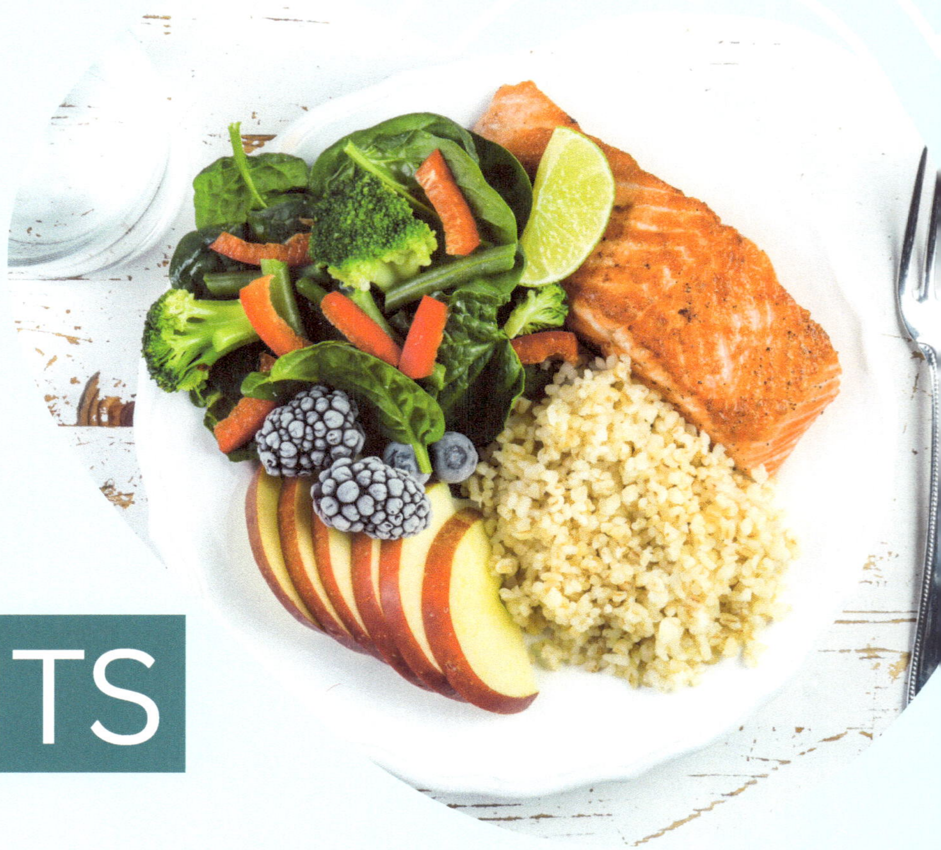

Get these important nutrients by eating a variety of healthy foods like vegetables and fruit, legumes (beans, lentils), seeds, grains, and fish. Protein helps to build muscle, which helps to keep bones strong. Although many foods contain calcium, dairy products provide the most calcium per serving size. Inadequate intake of nutrients increases the risk for bone loss and subsequent osteoporosis. Get your vitamin D everyday!

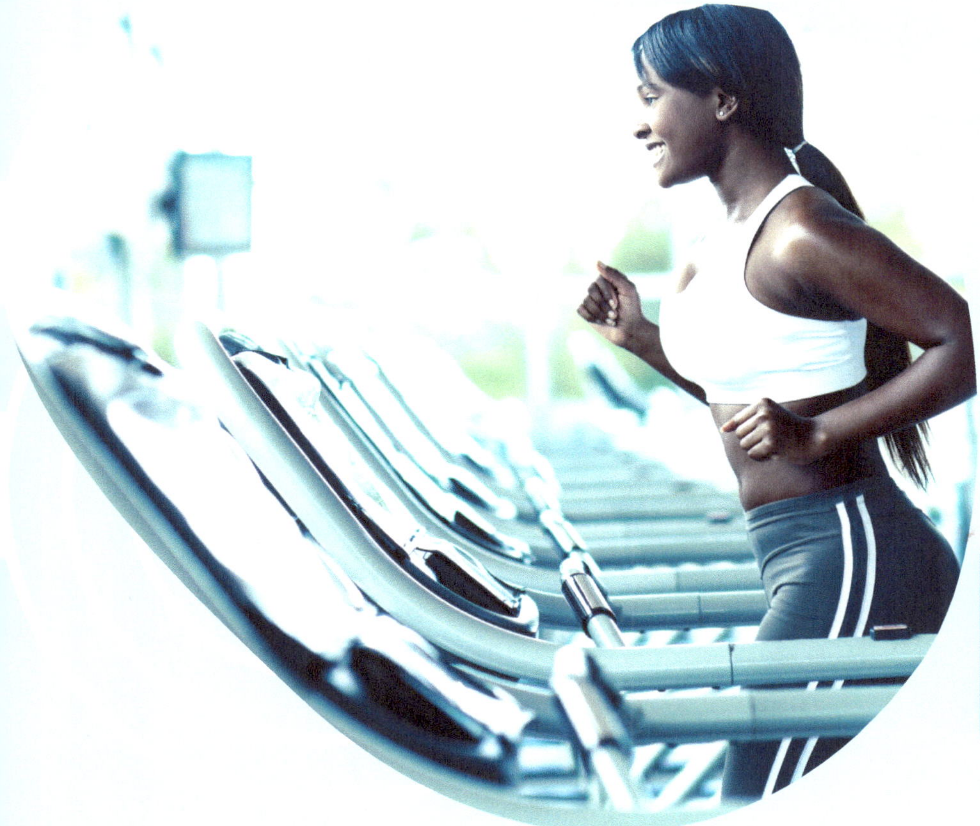

4 STAY ACTIVE

Aim to be active for at least 150 minutes each week. That's only 21 minutes a day. I know you can do more than that, however we'll make that the starting point. Here are some ideas to help keep your bones strong. Try:

- Weight-bearing exercises like walking, hiking, low impact aerobics, dancing, tennis and golf.
- Resistance activities like lifting weights or squats to help build muscle, which keeps your bones strong.

5 Limit CAFFEINE

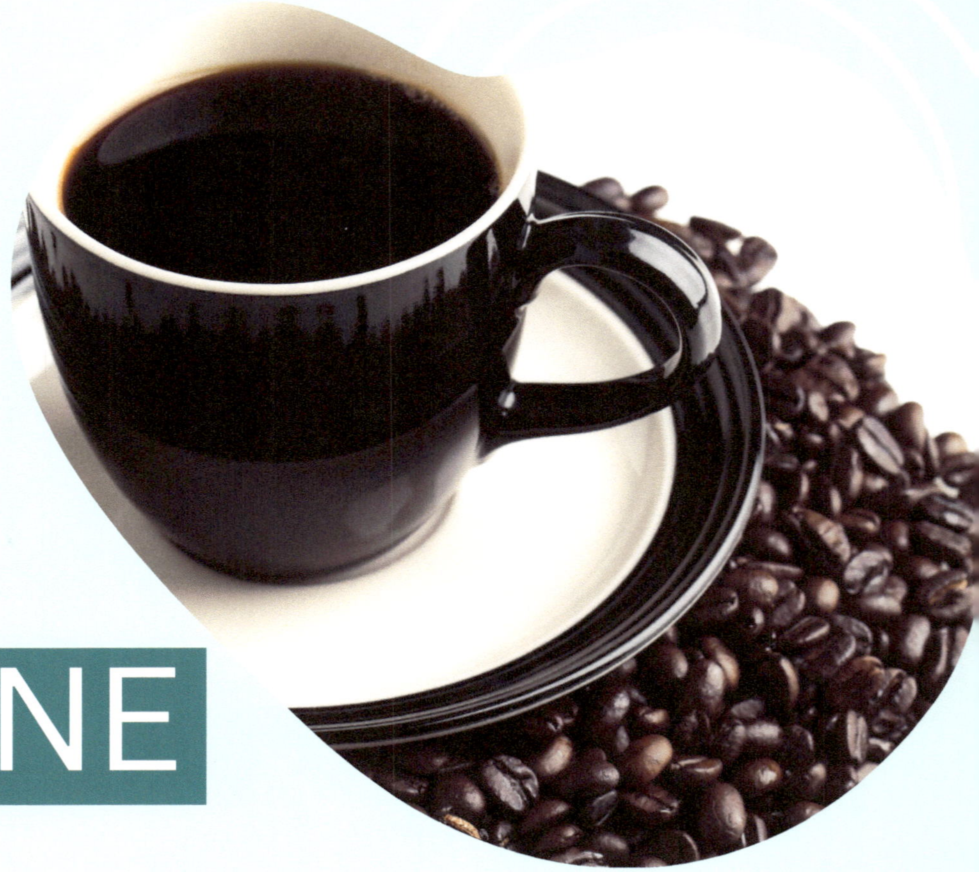

Having too much caffeine can decrease the amount of calcium you absorb. Too much caffeine intake can potentially create a calcium imbalance and inhibit bone formation. So in essence, caffeine leaches calcium from bones, sapping their strength. Black tea is excellent replacement for coffee. It can give you your caffeine fix with health benefits.

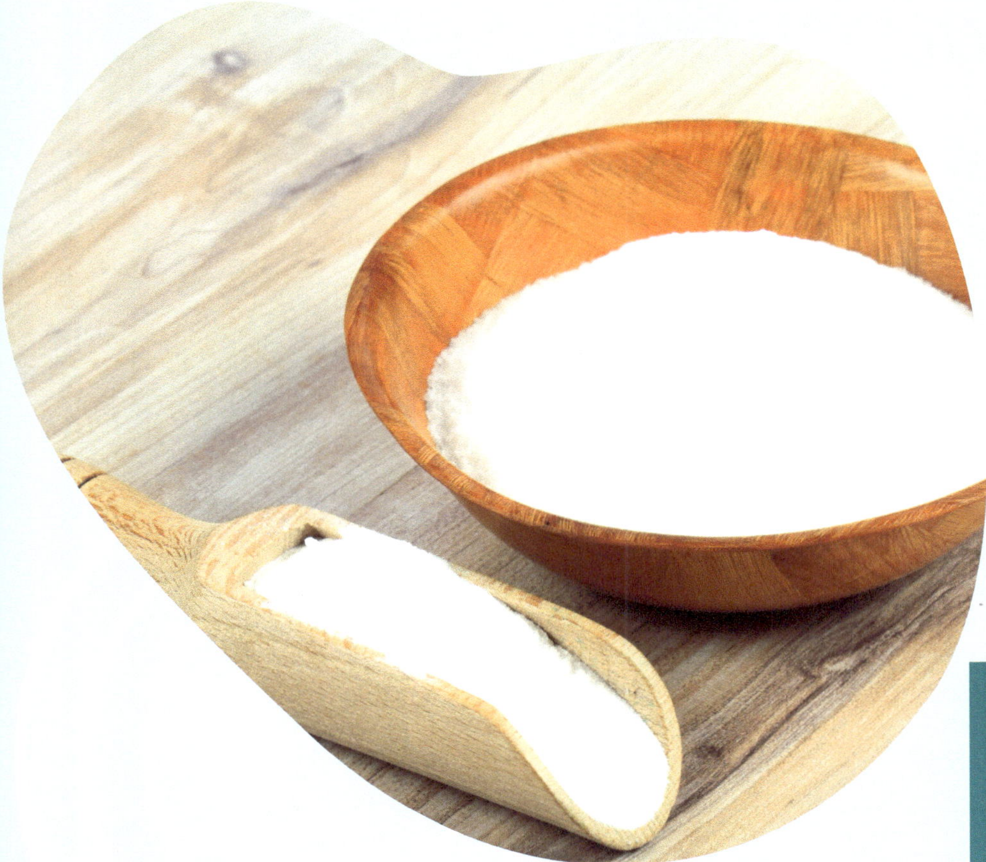

6

Don't Eat Too Much

SALT/ SODIUM

Too much sodium, which is found in salt, can reduce bone density. Salt is a major factor in controlling the amount of calcium in the urine and lost from the bones. Because calcium is important for bone strength, too much salt can lead to bone weakening and therefore may cause osteoporosis.

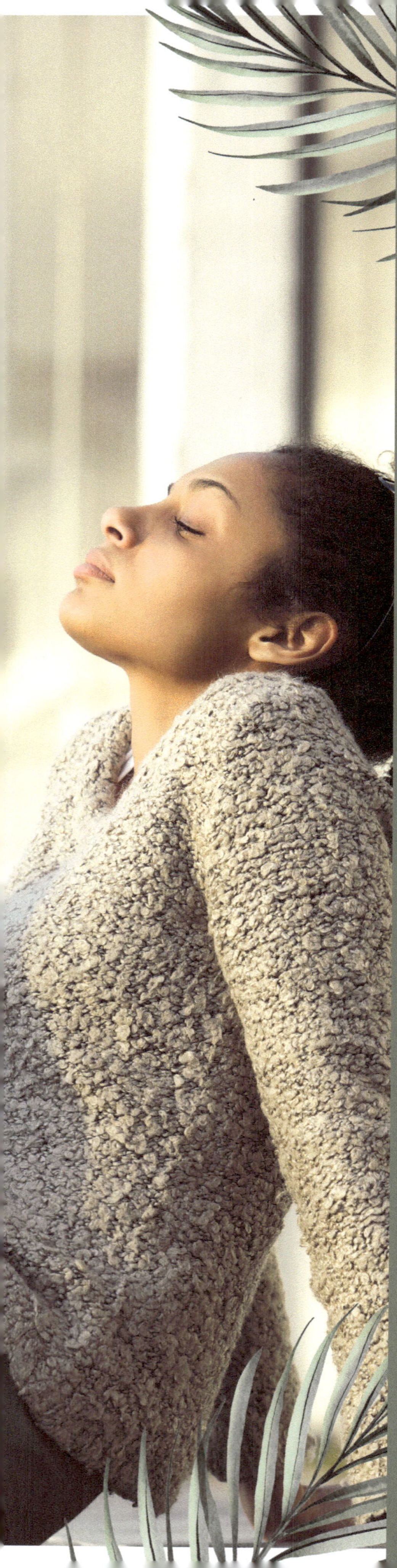

MENTAL HEALTH REMINDERS

1. Practice self-care
2. Connect with others
3. Stay active
4. Get enough sleep
5. Practice mindfulness
6. Eat a balanced diet
7. Seek support

FACTS

Most People Do Not Meet The Global Recommendation For Physical Activity

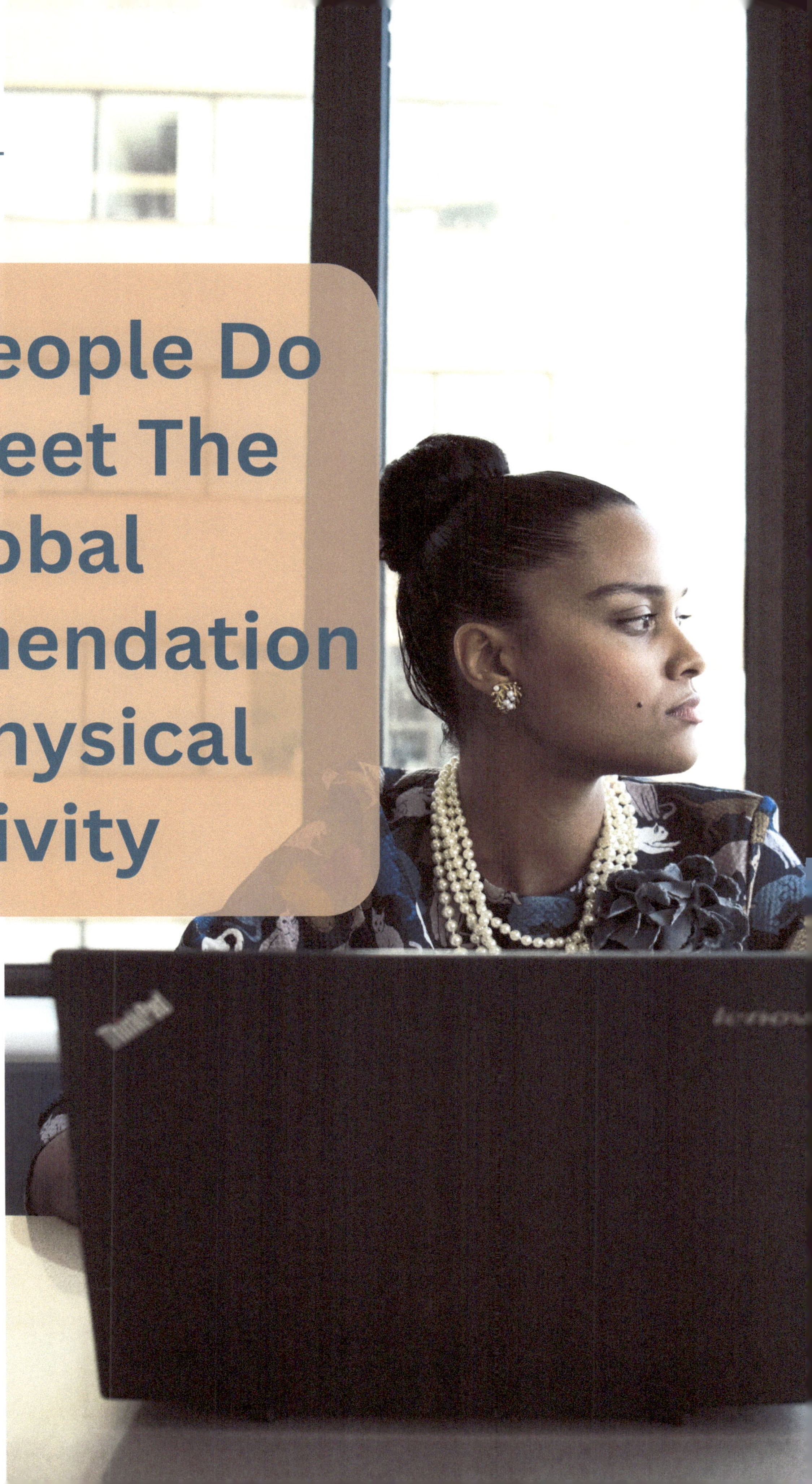

WHY IS DAILY ACTIVITY IMPORTANT?

We should aim to be active everyday as many ways as possible. The goal is to keep our circulatory system moving and our lymphatic system in motion. Our lymphatic system has a very important roll in keeping us healthy and ridding the body of cellular waste. It also keeps the body fluids balanced. This system of the body can not move on its own. The lymph fluid relies on the muscle movement of the body in order to get its job done. This means you, us, we, must move around!

When we get in our 30's our physical activity levels tend to slowly decrease but our mental stress increases. It is very important that once we turn 30 & beyond we make sure we incorporate daily physical activity.

ACTIVITY INTENSITY LEVELS

Moderate or vigorous activitity levels give you more energy and keeps your heart and lungs healthy. Moderate activity is when you can hold a conversation while performing the activity. Vigorous activity levels is when you can't say a few words without pausing to catch your breath.

You can incorporate moderate activities in your daily schedule and vigorous activity at least 3 times a week for no less than 30min cycles.

ACTIVITY OPTIONS

1

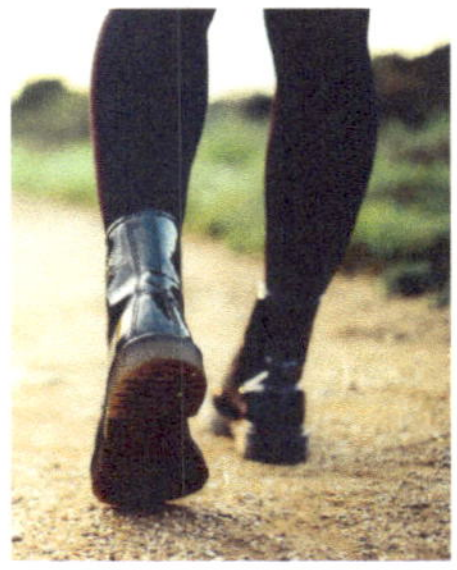

WALKING

Walking is the best exercise for the body. It reduces stress, gets your heart pumping, improves sleep, tones your muscles and more!

2

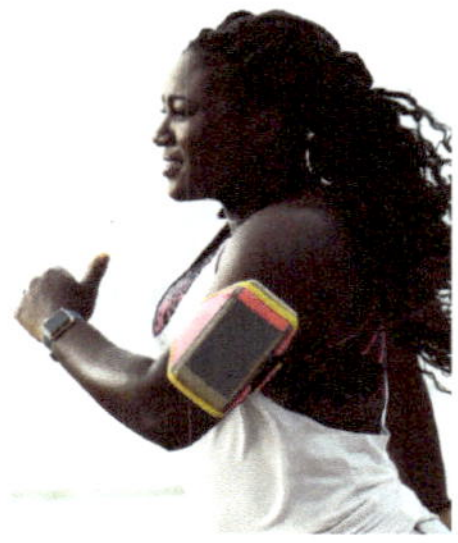

AEROBIC ACTIVITIES

This can be moderate or vigorous, just get the heart beating faster. Ex. swimming, cycling, household chores, gardening, jogging etc.

3

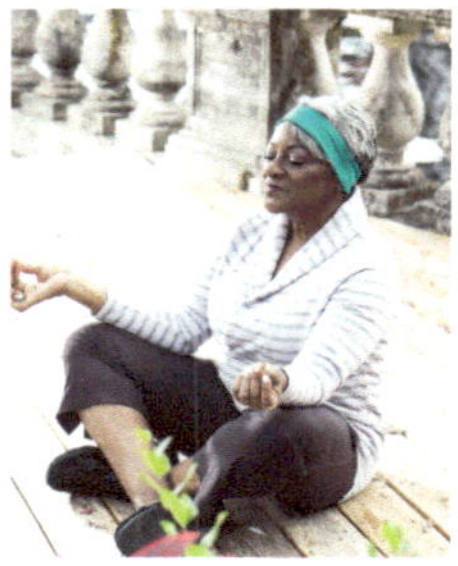

FLEXIBILITY

Relax those muscles and keep those joints mobile. Ex. dancing, yoga, pilates, weight training, walking, golf, stretching exercises etc,

4

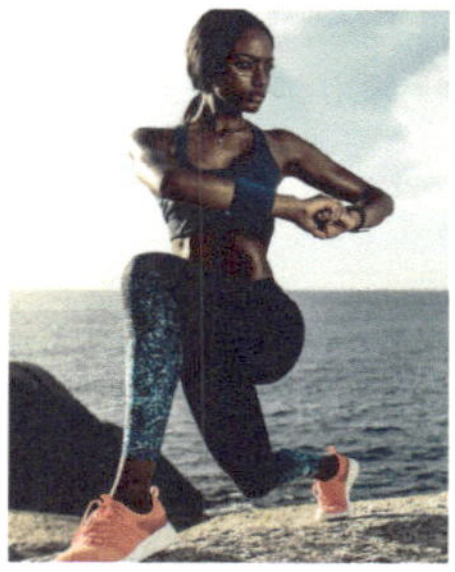

BALANCE

These activities are important to help us prevent falling. Ex. social dancing, chair raises, modified tai chi, bowling, yoga, etc.

5

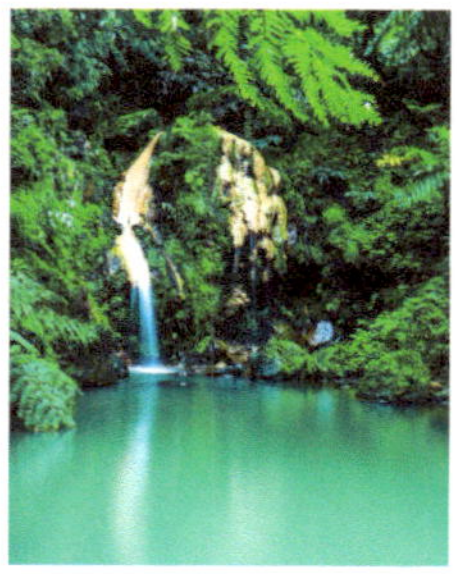

TRAVEL

Get away from your everyday normal scenery. Take a moment and disconnect from your ordinary life. Learn new cultures and experience other cuisines. Go camping or visit a safari! Enjoy life!

FREQUENTLY ASKED QUESTIONS

1 WHY IS MOVEMENT SO IMPORTANT?

Our bodies were created to be in motion. When we sit still for long periods of time we hurt various systems of the body. Here's a rule of thumb, for every hour sitting you should get up and walk around for 5 min. Take a walk outside to improve mental health and your immune system. Exercise also helps to lower stress levels and you don't have to go hard to receive the benefits.

2 HOW DO I DENTIFY WHEN FEELING TIRED IS SOMETHING I SHOULD BE CONCERED ABOUT?

Feeling fatigue can result from many things like stress, being overweight, having a poor diet, low iron, hormone imbalances and more. You should not feel tired all the time. If you do, the first thing you should do is make a doctors appointment and inform your physician. You should be concerned if you have poor concentration, you're yawning all day, you have tired or sore eyes, you feel restless and even experiencing slow response times to things.

3 UNEXPECTED WEIGHT GAIN IS TOO MUCH WHEN?

You should pay attention if **you put on weight without increasing your consumption of food or liquid and without decreasing your activity**. It could be due to fluid retention, abnormal growths, constipation, or pregnancy. This may also be due to menstruation, heart or kidney failure, preeclampsia, or medicines you take. You also might have swollen feet and ankles, a faster pulse, heavy breathing, high blood pressure, memory loss, and confusion. If this happens, contact your doctor.

4 WHAT TIME OF DAY IS BEST TO WORKOUT?

Ultimately it comes down to preference. Some can workout in the morning while others workout in the evenings and they both reap the same benefits. "Early workouts often lead to fewer distractions and increased productivity throughout the day", says Mark Brisby, a sports medicine doctor of chiropractic. While evening workouts may lead to better sleep and improved mood and concentration, make the decision according to what is needed in your life.

5 HOW LONG SHOULD I WAIT TO EAT AFTER A WORKOUT?

Eating within 30 minutes post-workout is ideal, but if possible, aim for within 1-2hrs. Protein is necessary to rebuild muscles, while carbs will re-stock glycogen, or energy stores, in your muscles.The best time to eat after a workout, in order to achieve weight loss, is within the first half hour after you're done exercising. That being said, keep in mind that weight loss really has to do with the amount you eat, more than when you eat it.

MEASURE YOUR INCHES NOT YOUR POUNDS

	DATE	DATE	DATE	DATE
NECK				
BICEPS				
CHEST				
WAIST				
UMBILICUS				
HIPS				
THIGHS				

MIND BODY CONNECTION EXERCISES

BOOST YOUR MENTAL

1

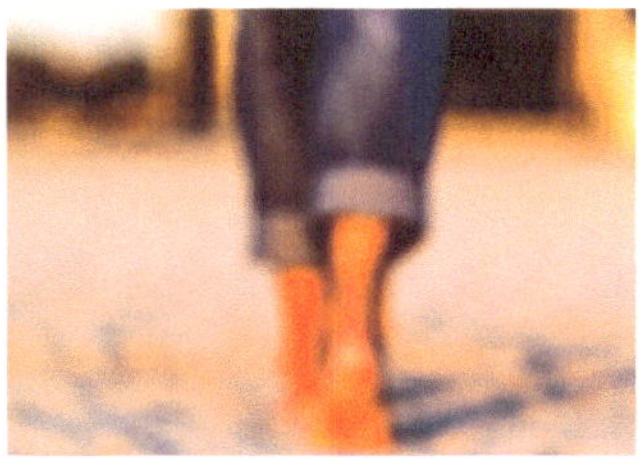

45

MINUTES

Walk outside in the sun.Enjoy nature! Look at the trees, water, grass, flowers, etc.

2

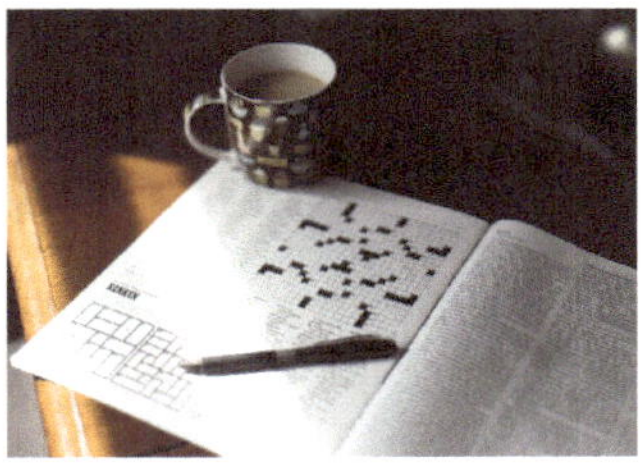

0

NO TIME LIMIT

Sit down and do a crossword or jigsaw puzzle. It relaxes and grows brain power all at the same time.

3

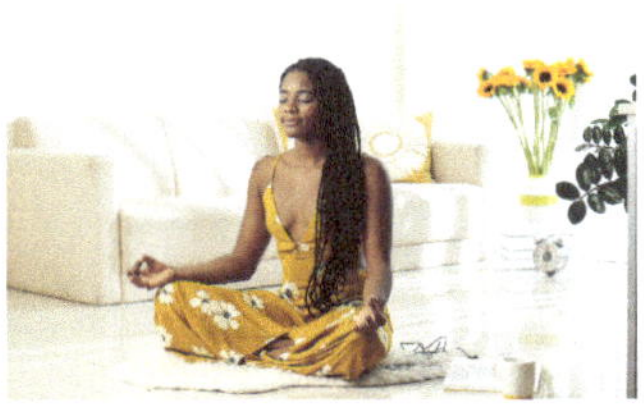

30

MINUTES

Meditation provides the body with a sense of calmness, it releases stress & provides balance.

4

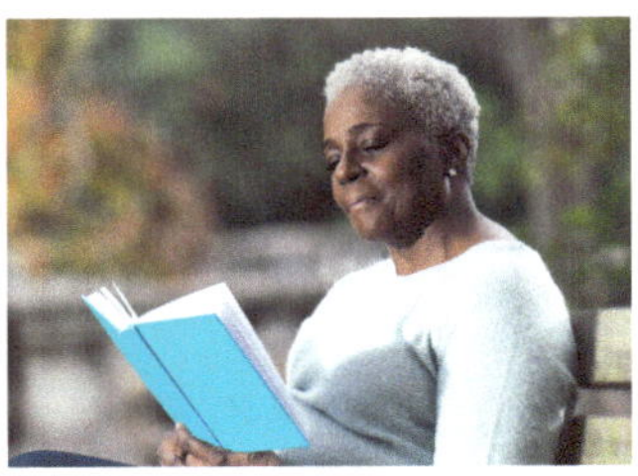

5

TIMES
A WEEK

Reading improves connections in the brain. It improves concentration & memory.

5

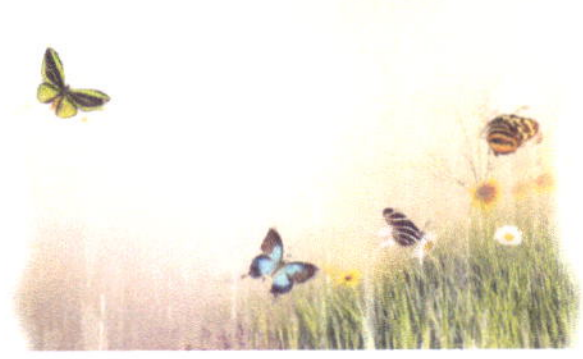

1

A WEEK

Painting or coloring enhances brain functions. Not just doing them but also looking at them.

6

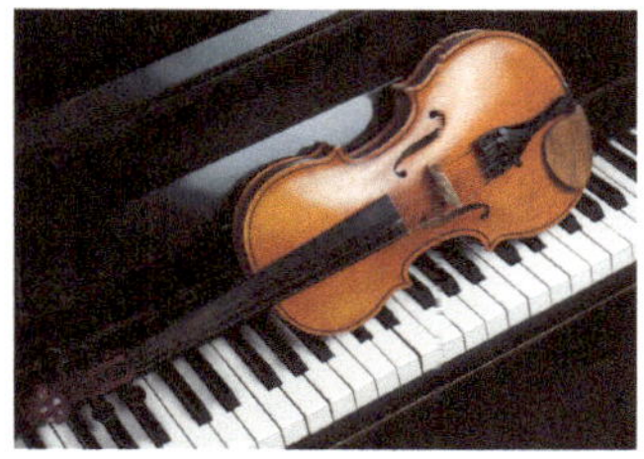

0

NO TIME LIMIT

Learn a new skill. The brain benefits when we learn a new language or how to play an instrument.

7

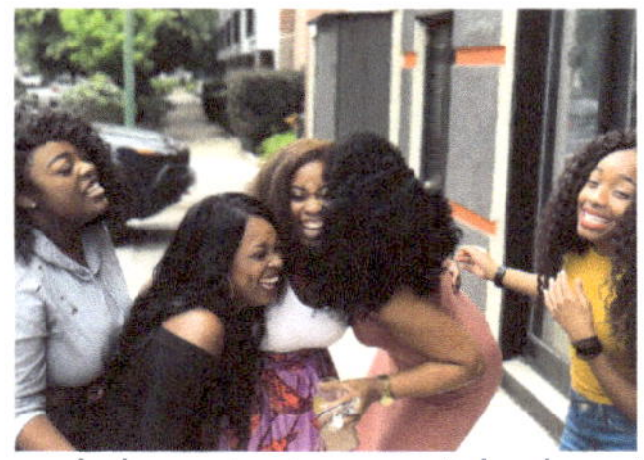

1

DAILY

Positive social engagement helps to repair the damaging effects of stress. It activates the reward system of the brain.

8

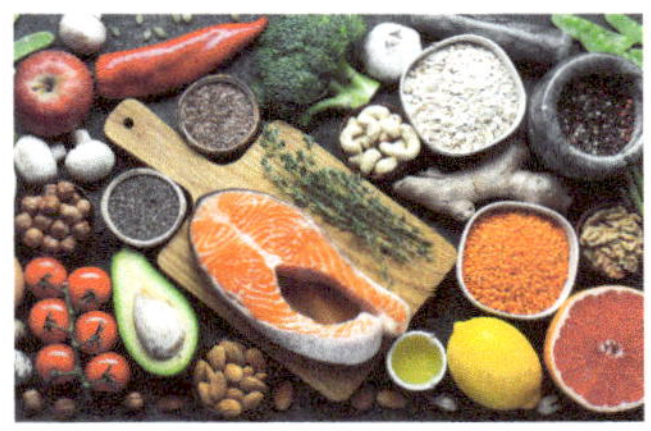

1

DAILY

Making healthy food choices reduces mood swings and increases the ability to focus.

9

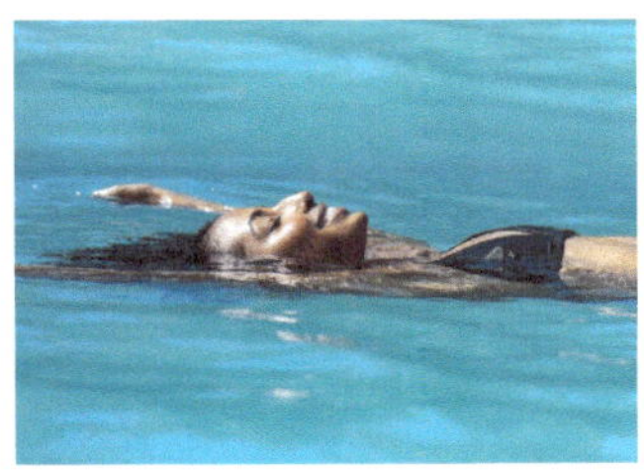

0

NO LIMIT

Swimming releases endorphins in the brain, your feel good hormones. The water increases the sense of wellbeing.

10

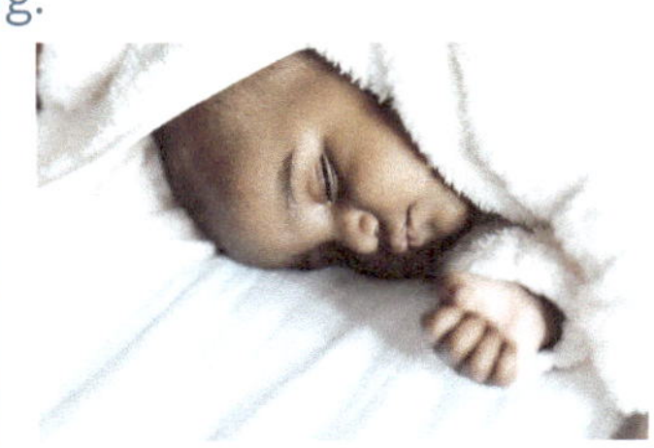

1

DAILY

Without the proper rest we can not form or maintain pathways in our brains. Sleep like a baby.

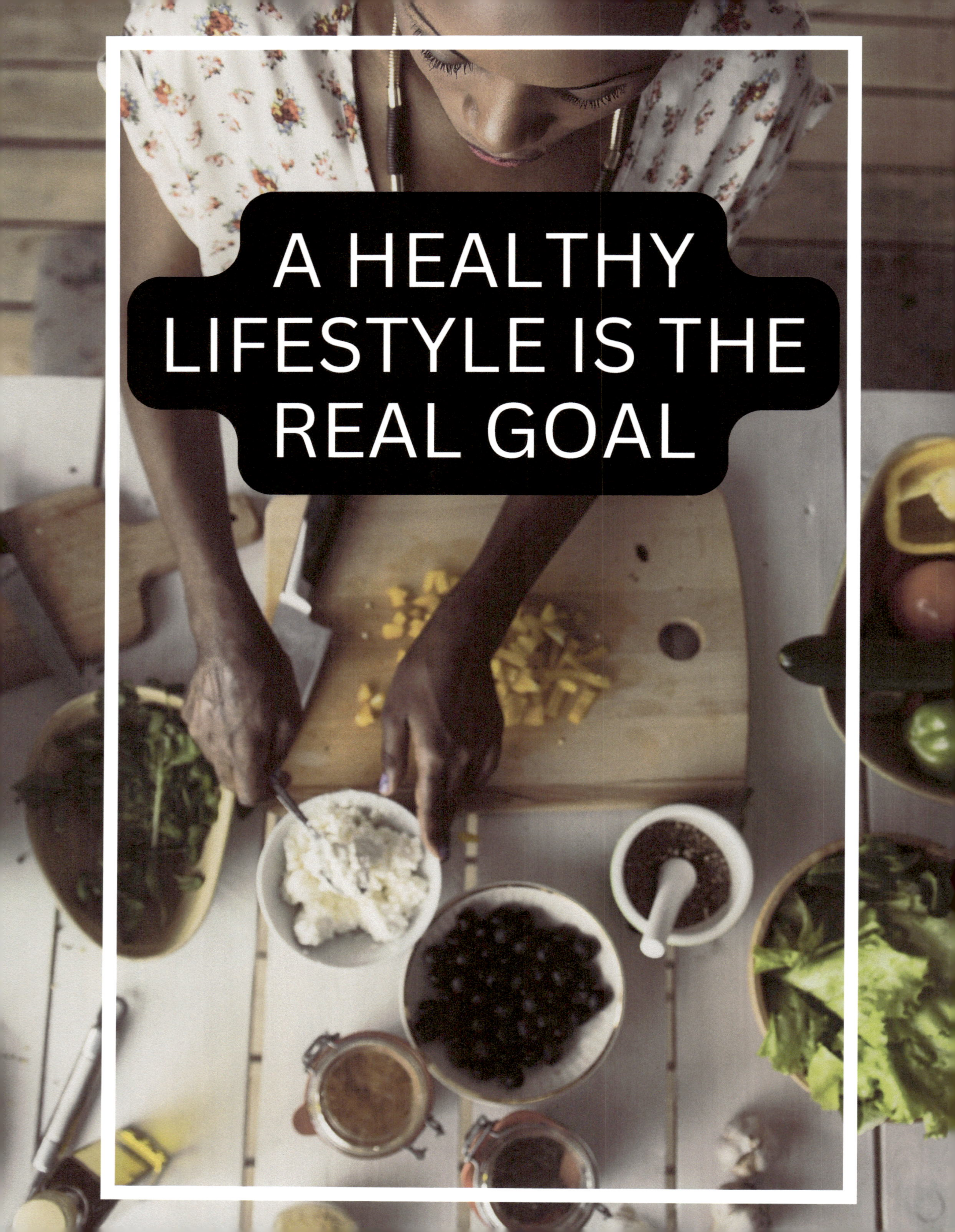
A HEALTHY LIFESTYLE IS THE REAL GOAL

Benefits Of

Writing A Journal Or A Diary

Set & attain your objectives

Enhance your writing skills

Boost Your Memory

Record ideas on-the-go

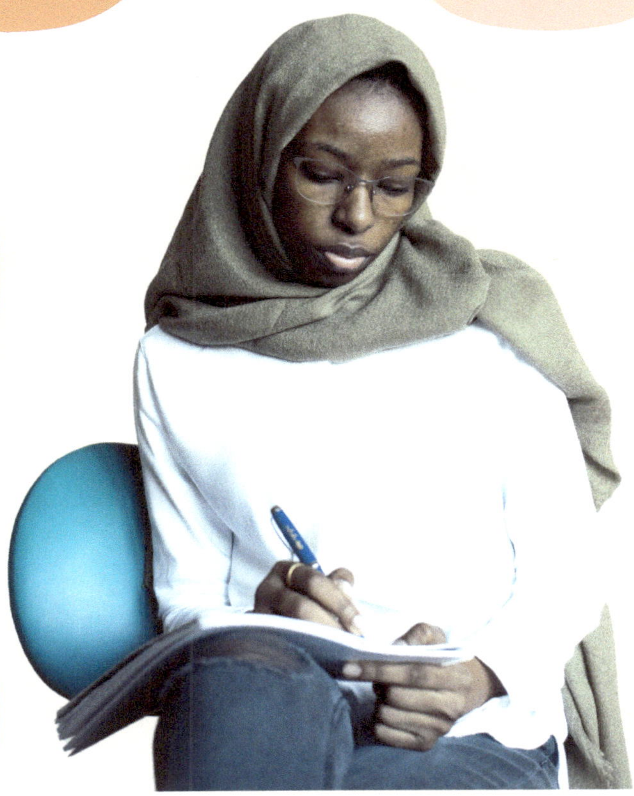

Keep your thoughts organized

Relieve Stress

Self-Reflection Questions

What is one goal in life? ____________________

What is one of my strengths? ____________________

What do I love about myself? ____________________

Who matters the most to me? ____________________

What am I ashamed of? ____________________

What do I like to do for fun? ____________________

What am I worried about? ____________________

Where do I feel safest? ____________________

Who gives me comfort? ____________________

Who is my happiest memory with? ____________________

What keeps me grounded? ____________________

What am I grateful for? ____________________

What are my values? ____________________

When am I at my best? ____________________

What brings me joy? ____________________

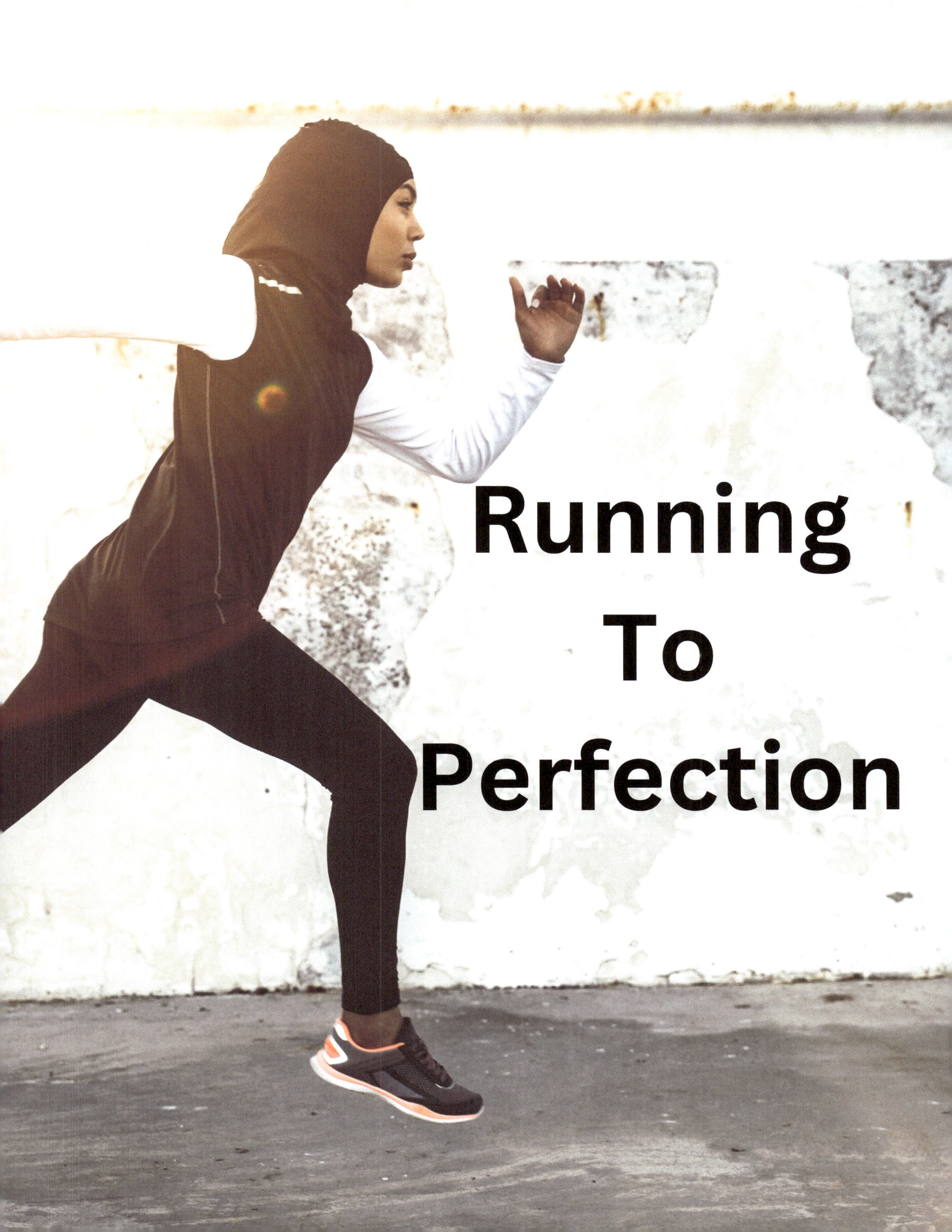

Running To Perfection

PINEAPPLE CRANBERRY SMOOTHIE

Yields 2

¾ cup Cranberry Juice

¾ cup frozen pineapple chunks

½ frozen banana

1 (5.3-oz) container light vanilla Greek yogurt

½ teaspoon vanilla extract (optional)

1 T raw organic honey (optional)

Place cranberry juice, pineapple, banana, and Greek yogurt in blender. Blend until smooth. Serve immediately.

NOTE: If the smoothie is too tart, you can add the vanilla and honey to sweeten it a bit.

* Frozen banana makes the smoothie a little thicker, but you can use a non-frozen banana.

PINA COLADA PROTEIN SMOOTHIE

Yields 1

1 cup unsweetened vanilla almond milk

¾ cup frozen pineapple chunks

1 scoop vanilla protein powder

1 teaspoon raw honey

1 teaspoon vanilla

Place almond milk, pineapple, vanilla protein powder, honey, and vanilla in blender.

Blend until smooth. Serve immediately.

Recipes from halfscratched.com

THREE INGREDIENT SMOOTHIE

Not all healthy smoothies require a lot of ingredients. Here are a few that doesn't take much to whip up. ***Add ice to all recipes.***

Cantaloupe

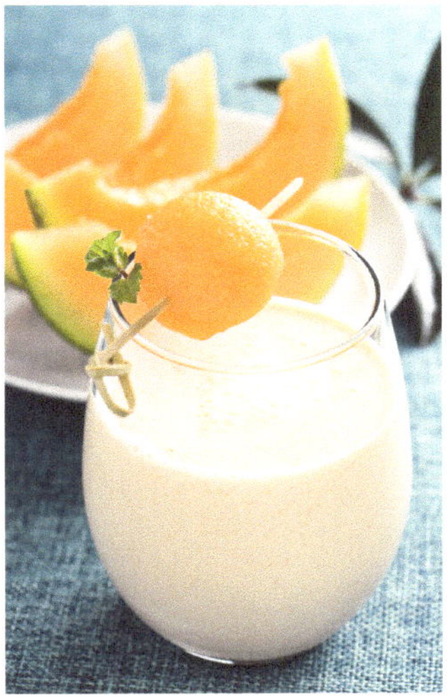

=

Vanilla Yogurt 1 cup

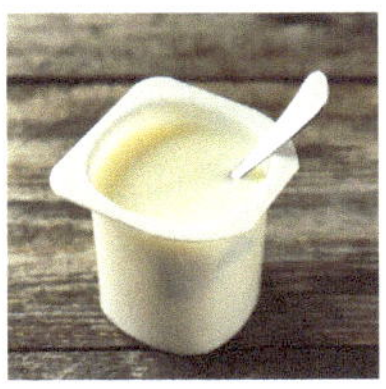

+

1/2 cup of orange juice

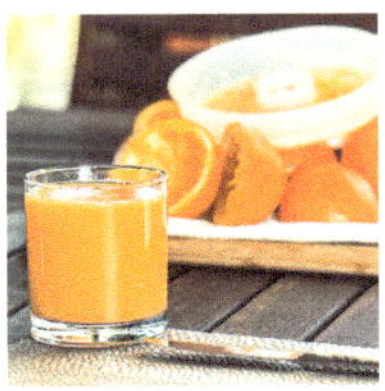

+

1/2 cup of sliced cantaloupe

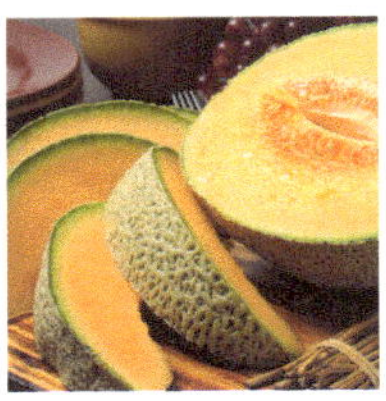

Mango Cherry

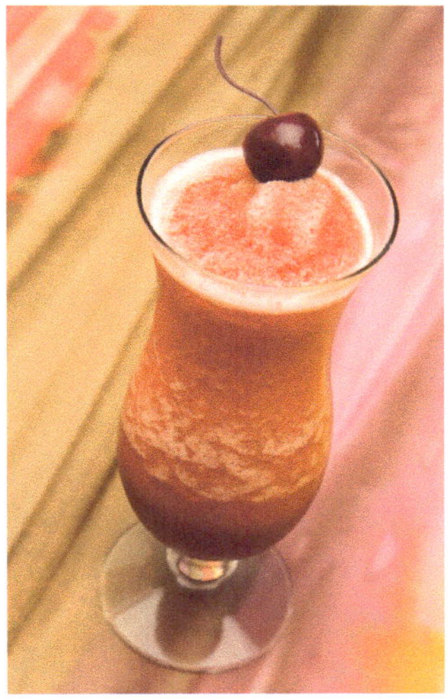

=

2 cups of cherries

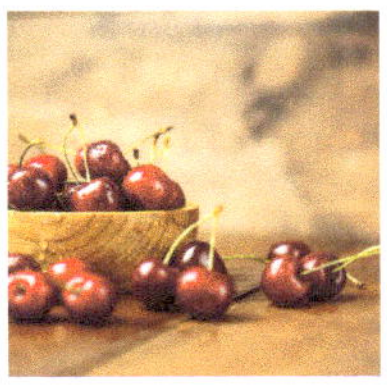

+

1 cup of chopped mango

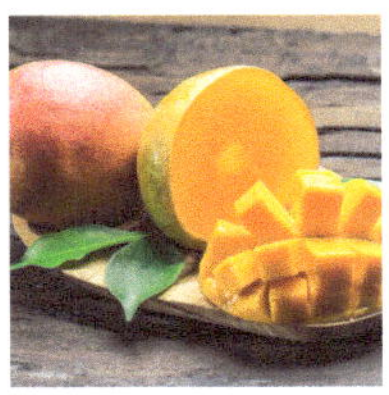

+

1 cup of water

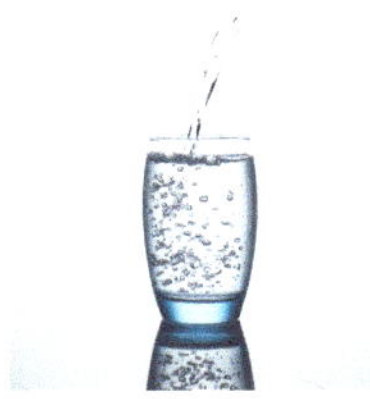

Strawberry Banana

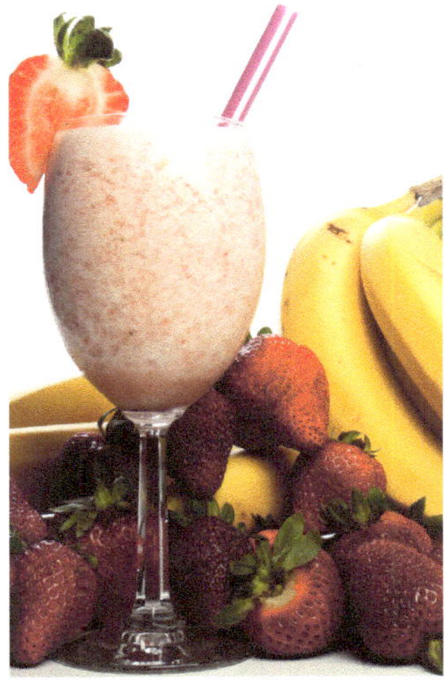

=

1 ripe banana sliced

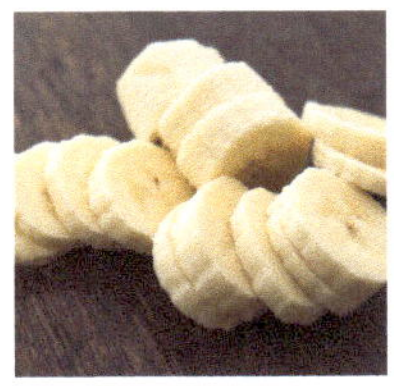

+

10oz of fresh straw-berries

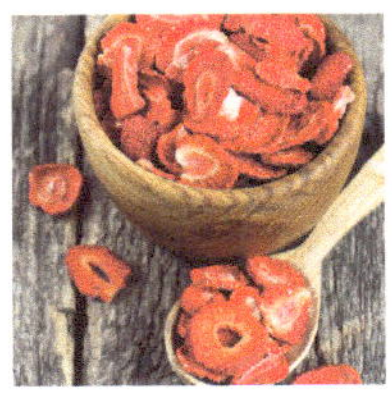

+

1/2 cup of milk

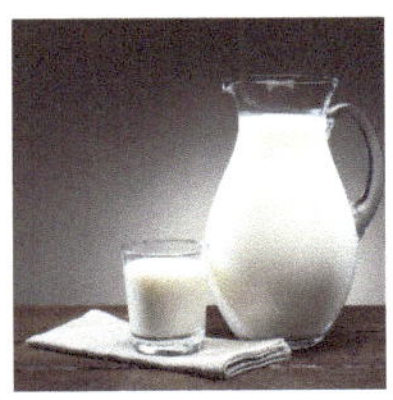

Blend smoothie recipes until smooth or your desired thickness.

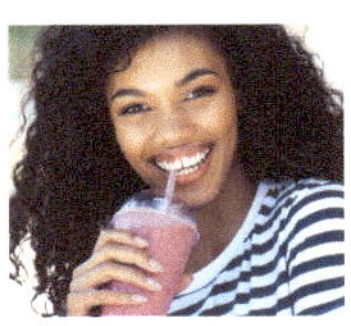

Cucumber Benefits For Your Body

Prevents dehydration

Fights free radicals

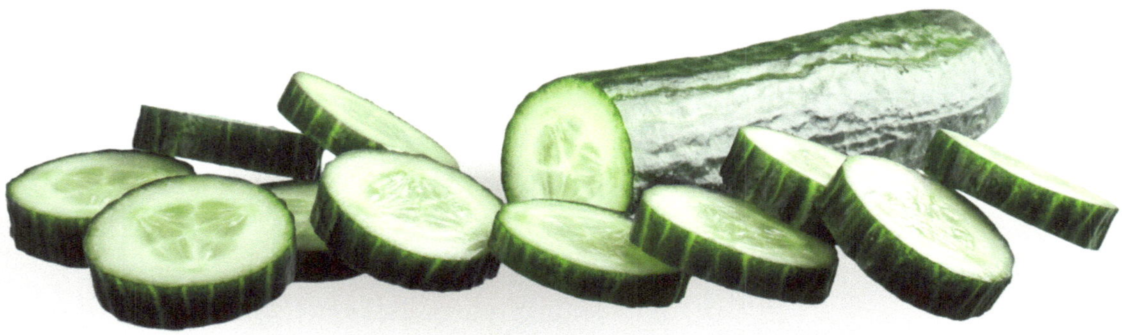

Maintains healthy skin

Smoothens digestion

Helps lose weight

BENEFITS OF FRUIT
& its contents

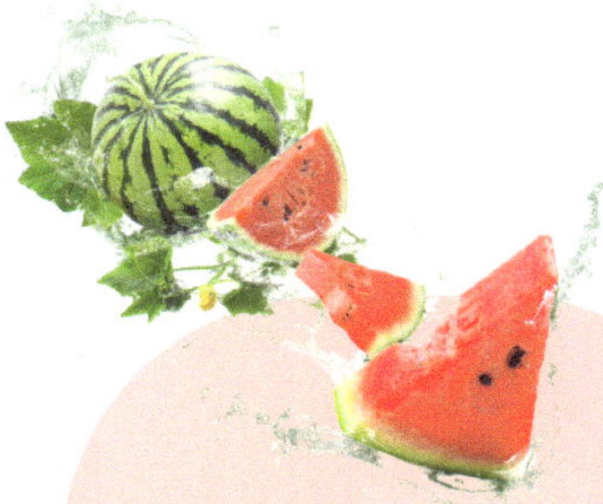

Watermelon

Watermelon contains vitamin A & C and the antioxidant lycopene. Watermelon can prevent dehydration and is good for heart health.

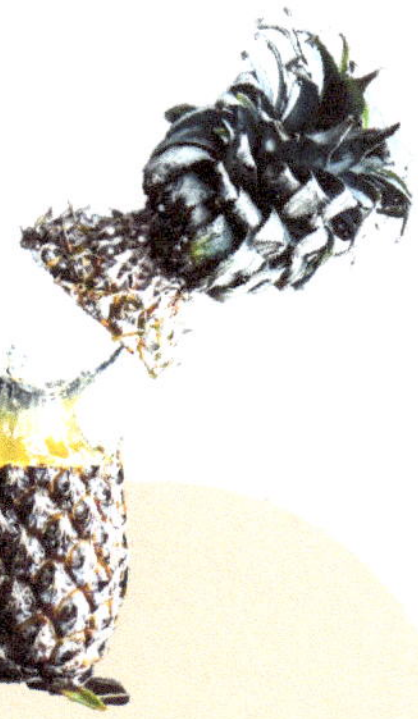

Pineapple

Pineapple is rich in antioxidants and contains vitamin C which is good for increasing endurance and preventing various diseases.

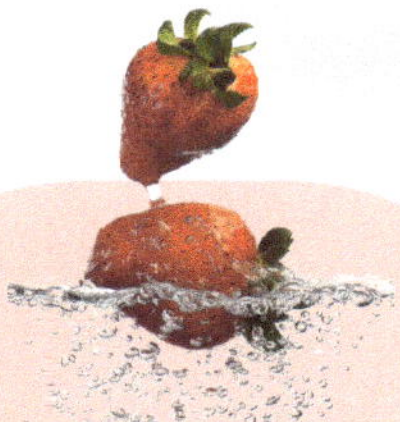

Strawberry

Strawberries contain vitamin C and are rich in antioxidants, which are helpful in reducing the growth of cancerous cells.

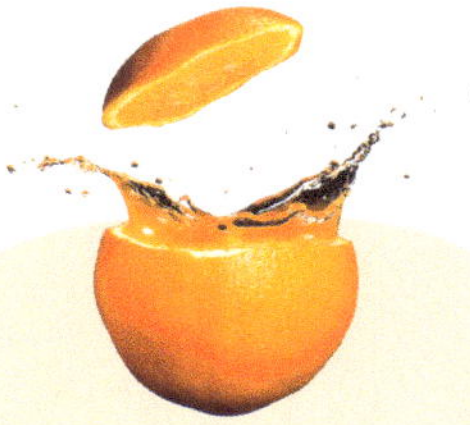

Orange

Oranges are a source of vitamin C, contain vitamin B1, folate, and potassium which are useful for boosting the body's immunity.

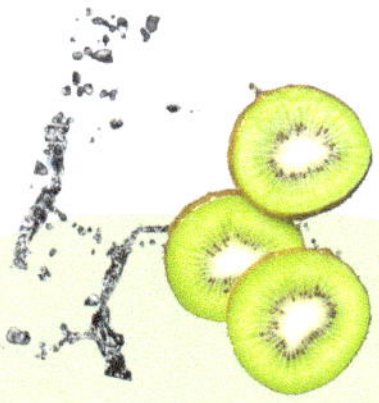

Kiwi

The content of vitamin C in kiwi fruit is beneficial for skin health, can prevent premature aging and overcome acne.

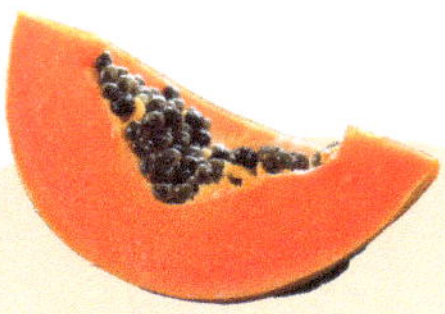

Papaya

Papaya contains two proteolytic enzymes, papain and chymopapain, which is helpful for protein digestion and helps digestive problems.

Health Benefits Of

Cayenne Pepper

Increases the production of digestive fluid, sends enzymes to the stomach to aid in digestion, and provides extra protection to the stomach against infections.

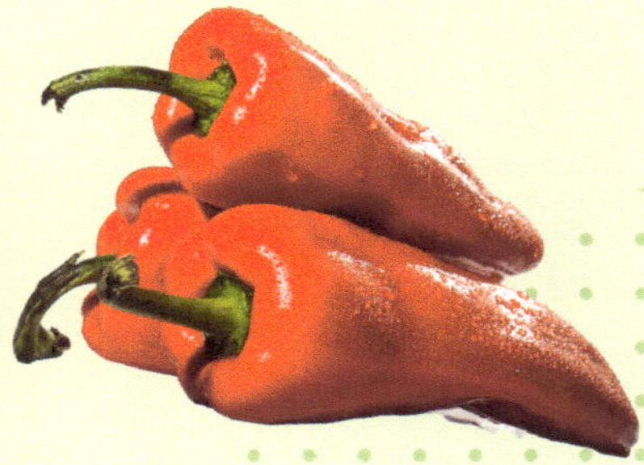

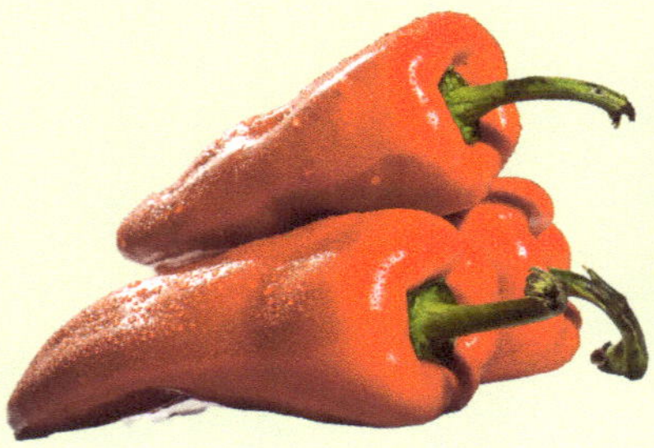

It makes the perfect detoxifier, helping to flush toxins from the body, while stimulating circulation and neutralizing acidity in the body.

Reduces the risk of liver inflammation.

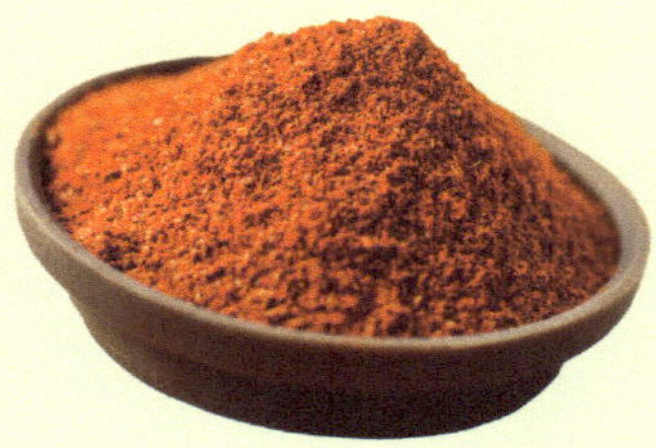

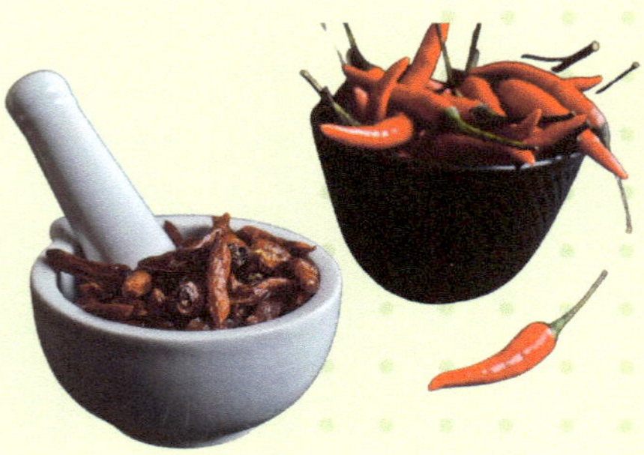

It helps keep blood pressure under control and may help reduce kidney stones and bone loss as you age.

Health Benefits Of

HONEY

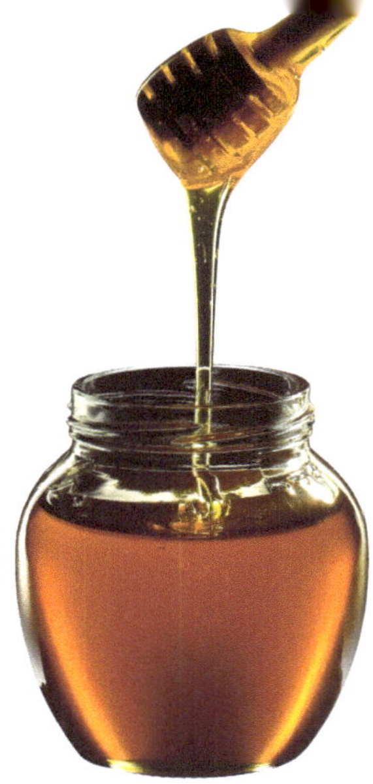

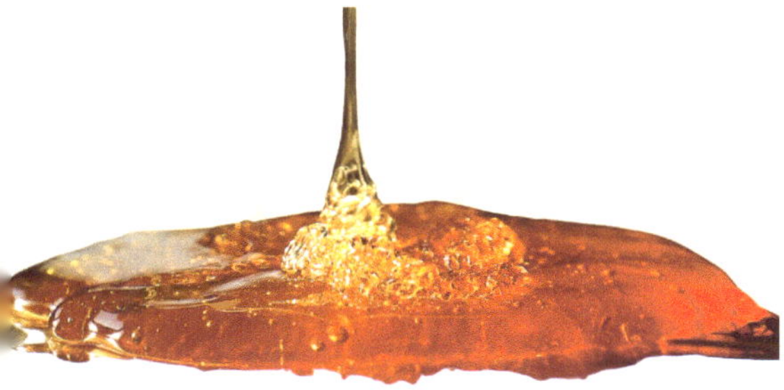

Counteract free radicals

Increase body immunity

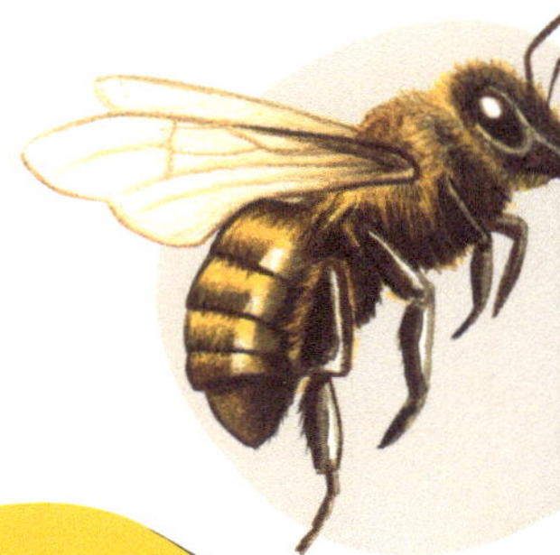

Help to relieve coughs

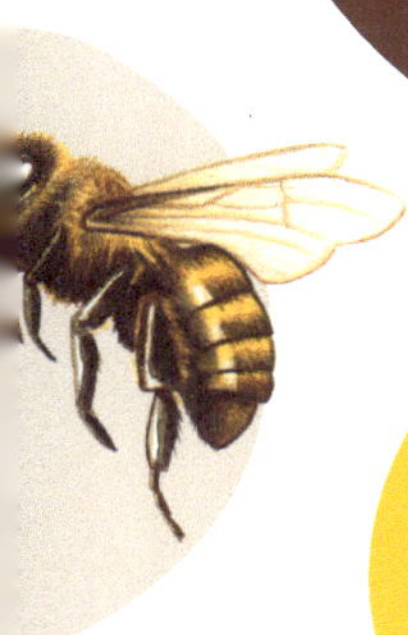

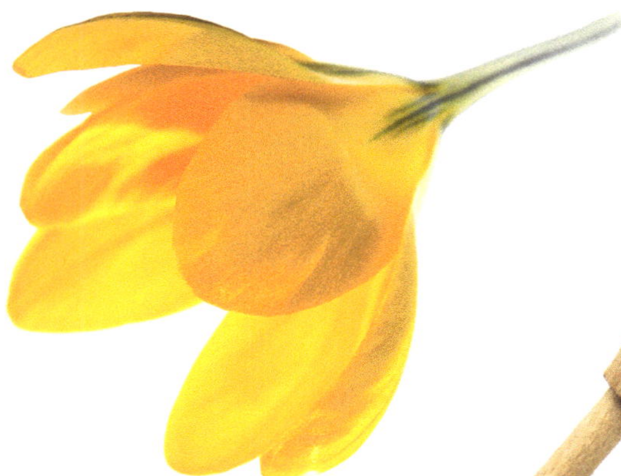

Energy booster

Lower blood pressure

Maintain cholesterol levels

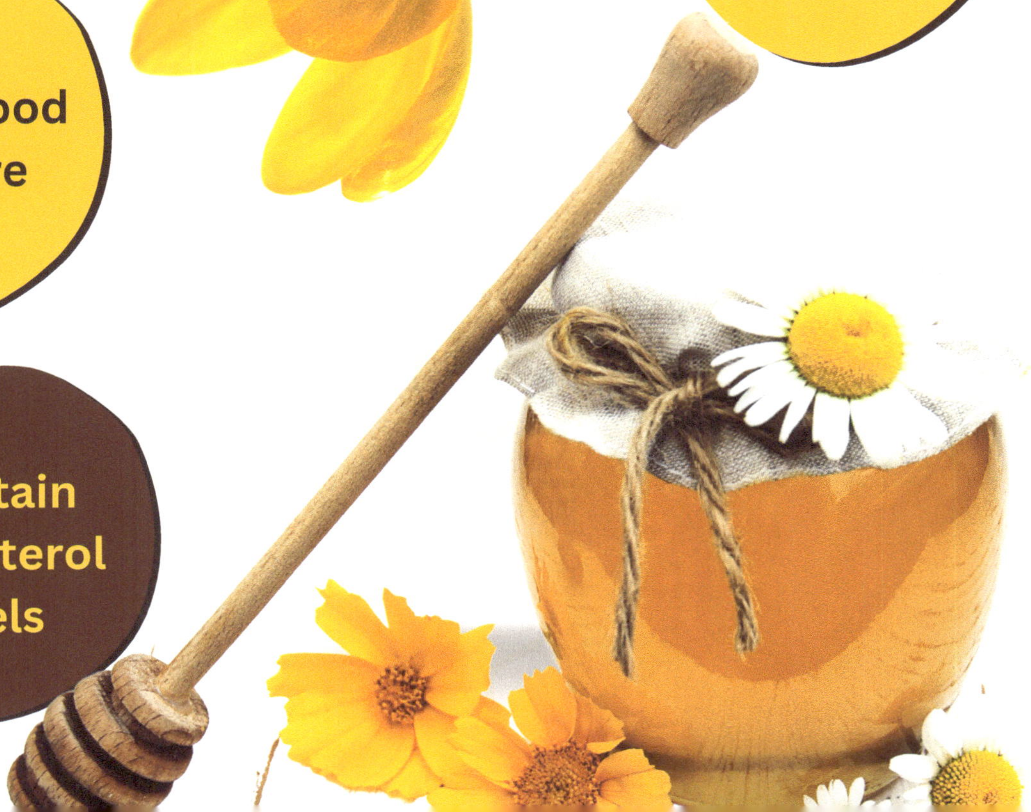

Benefits of
Vitamin A For Health

Maintain eye health

Maintain healthy reproductive organs

Strengthen the immune system

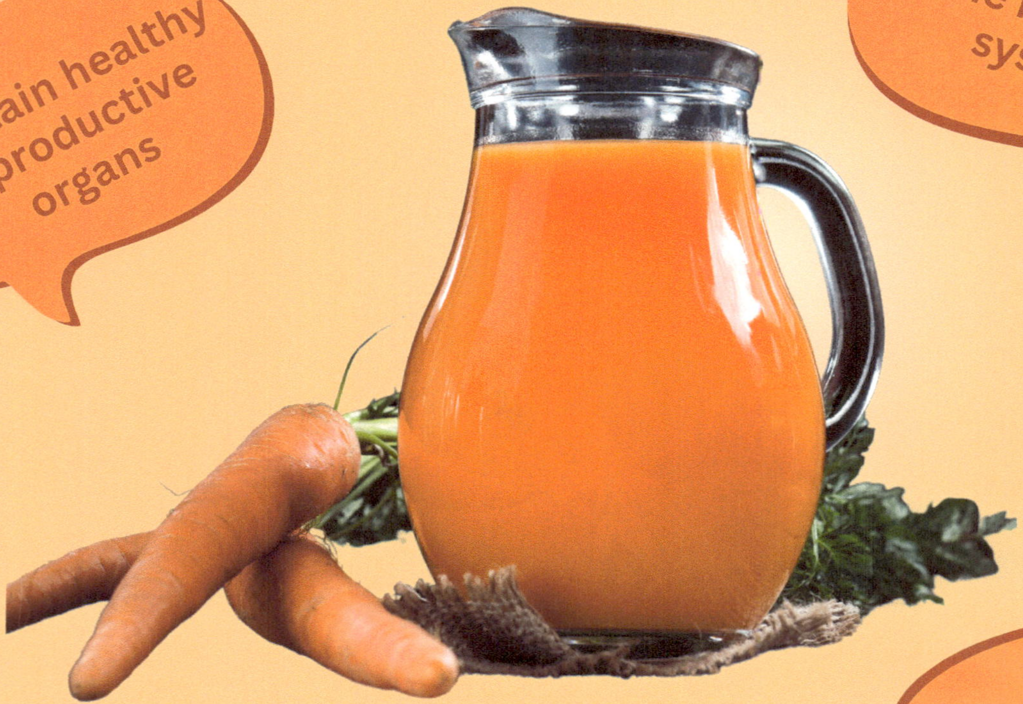

Helps bone health

Helps to produce red blood cells

Reduce the growth of pimples

Why is fiber good for you?

Can help you lose weight

You'll have a lower chance of contracting a number diseases

Makes your gut bacteria happy

Help reduce constipation

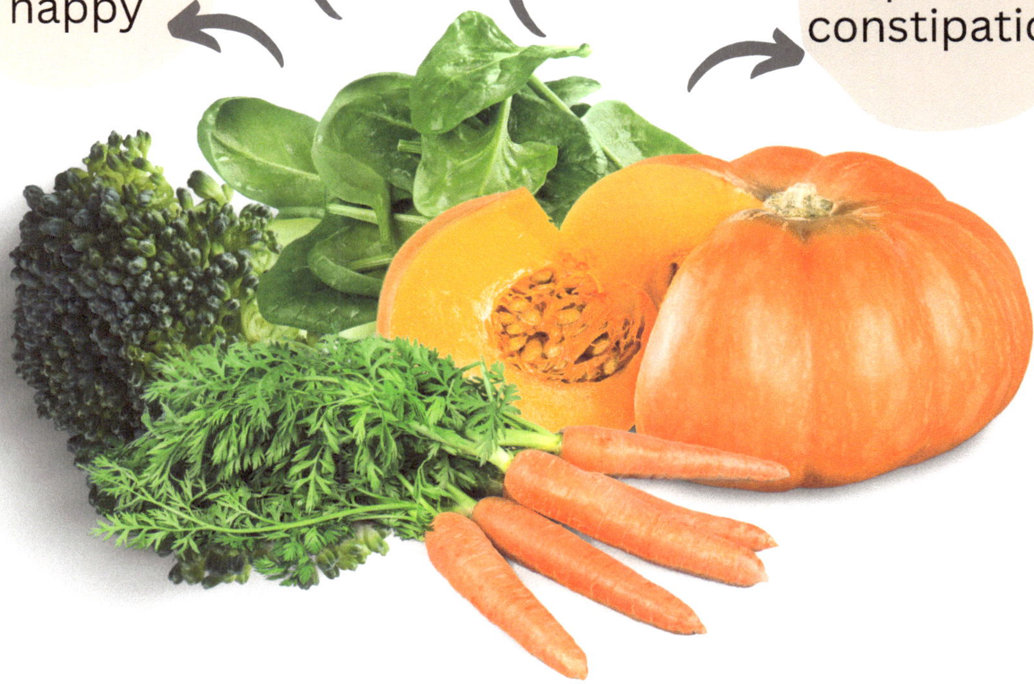

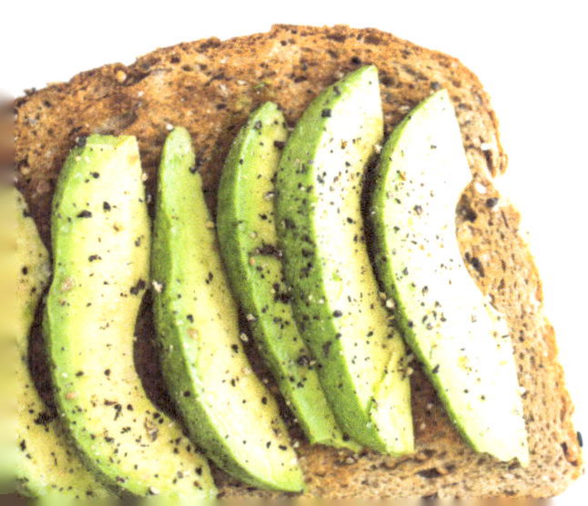

HIGH FIBER

BENEFITS OF *Activated Charcoal* FOR YOUR HEALTH

- Whitens Your Teeth
- Helps You Get Clearer Skin, Smaller Pores, & Less Oil
- Volumizes Hair & Reduces Dandruff
- Improves Acne Issues
- A Gentle Exfoliator

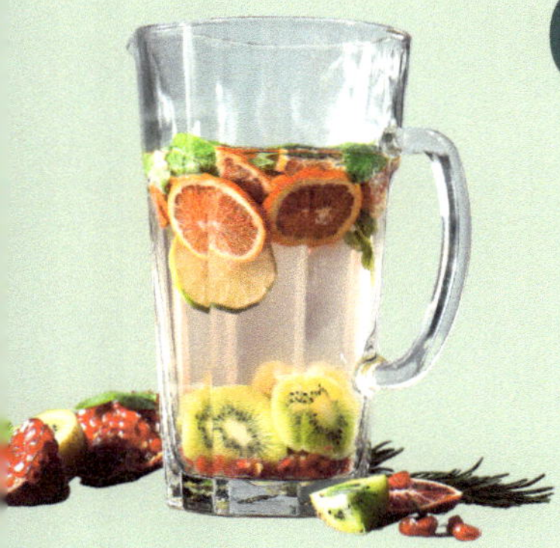

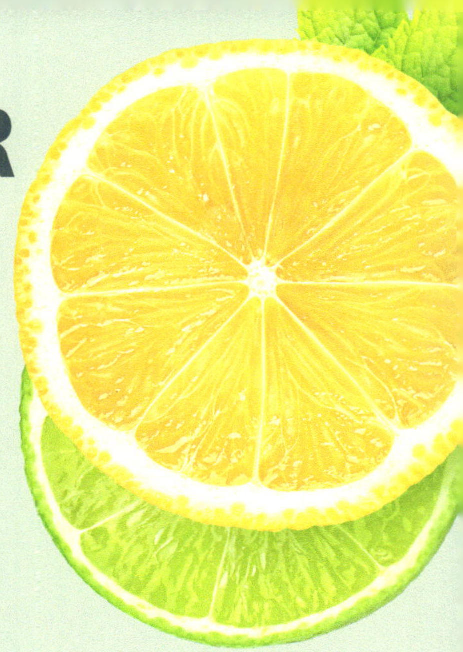

INFUSED WATER OPTIONS & ITS BENEFITS

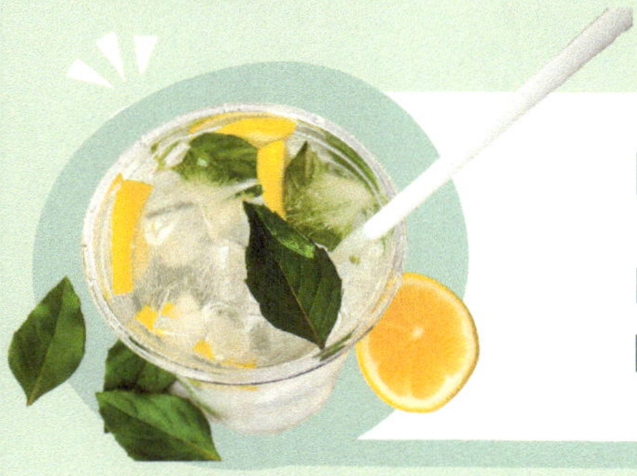

Lemon + Basil leaves

Reduces inflammation and prevents kidney stones.

Lime + Ginger:

Helps your blood circulation to be better and make your skin healthier.

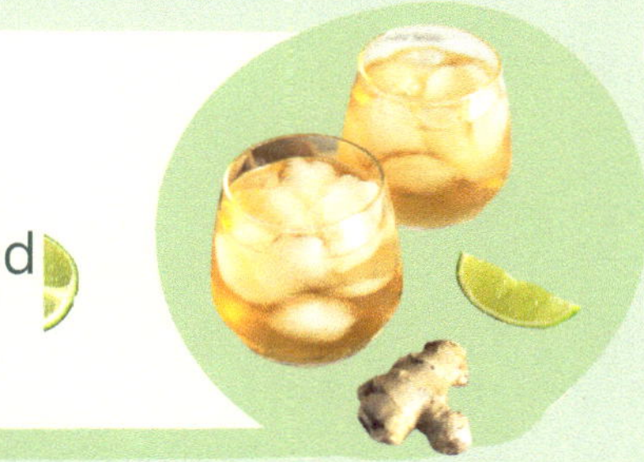

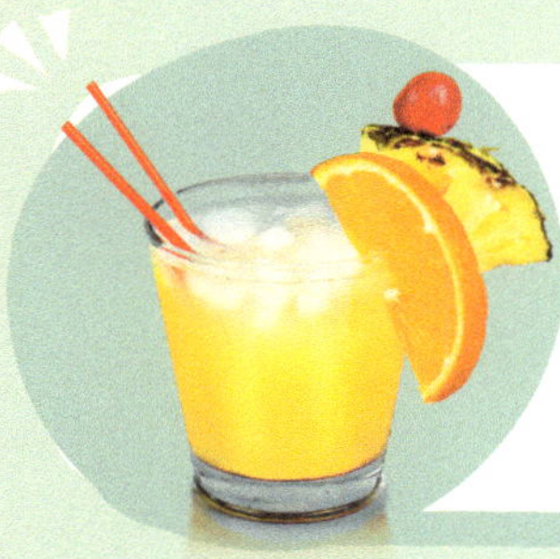

Pineapple + Orange:

Contains a high level of Vitamin C and boosts your immune system.

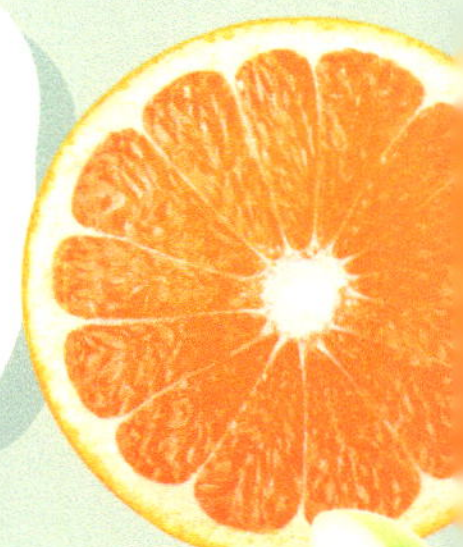

Apple + Cinnamon:

Supports your digestive organs and lowers the risk of getting diabetes or heart disease.

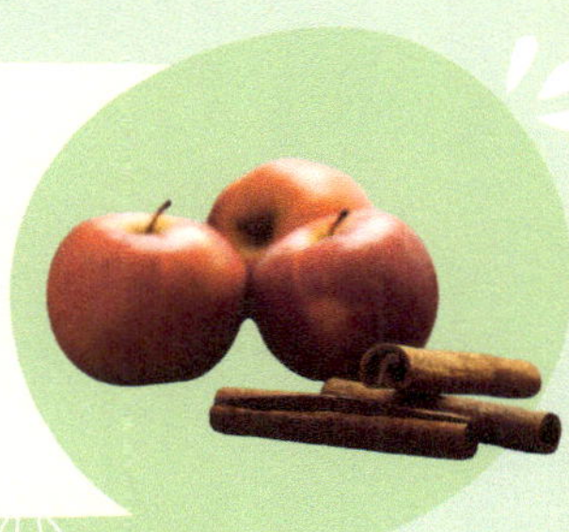

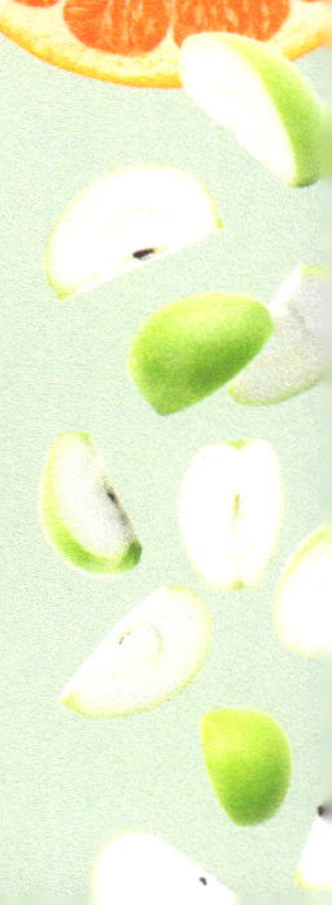

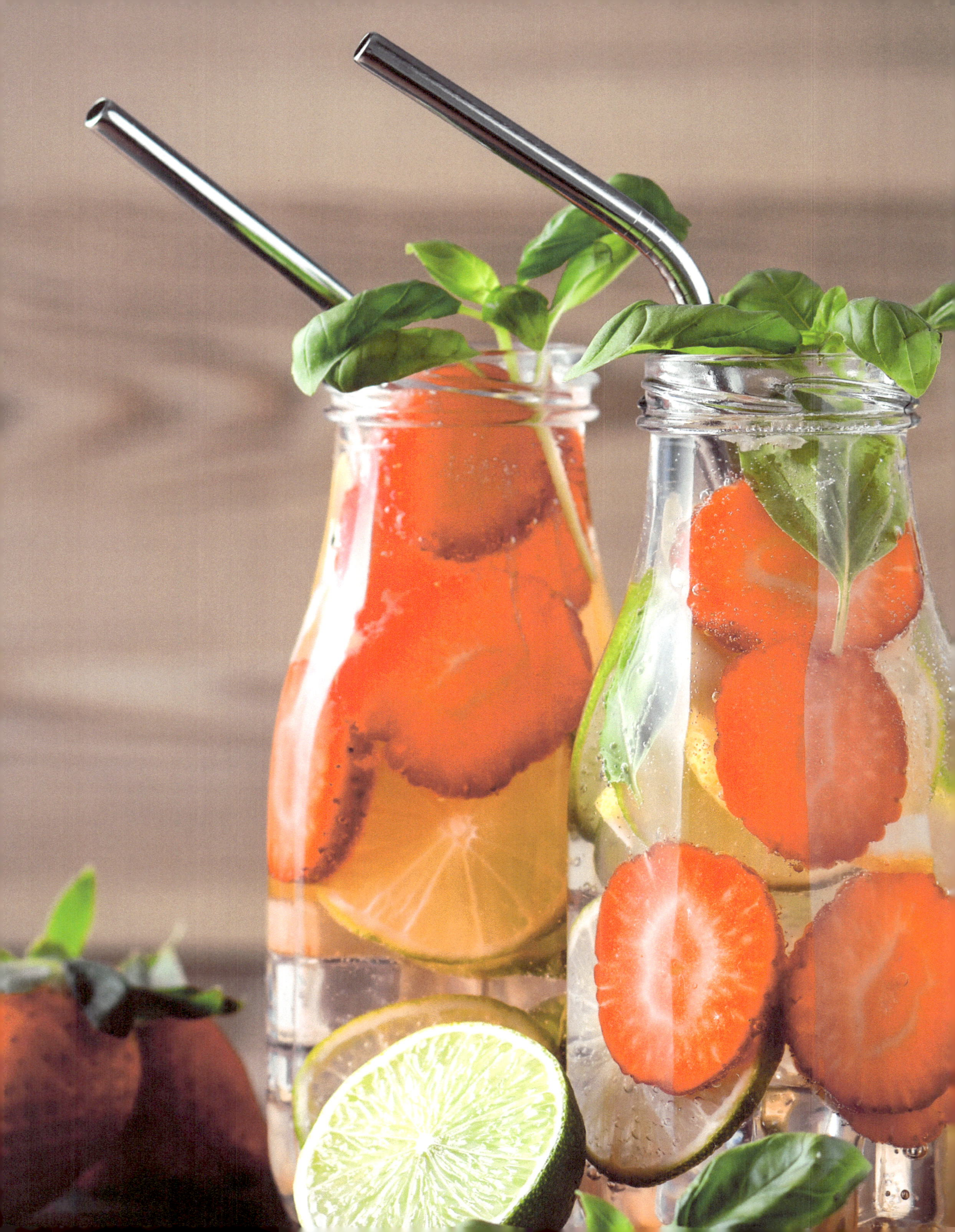

STRAWBERRY INFUSED WATER

Ingredients

24oz of Water
Fresh Organic Strawberries
Fresh Organic Limes
Fresh Organic Lemons
Freash Organic Mint Leaves
Ice

Instructions

Wash the fruits and mint leaves thoroughly.
Next, cut up strawberries into halves
Cut up lemons & limes into circular pieces.
You can leave mint leaves whole.
Fill up your desired container full of water
(leaving room for ice to be added).
Place all the sliced fruit into the water and add ice to the top.
Refrigerate for at least 24 hours to allow fruits to be infused in the water.
Enjoy your delicious infused Water!

D

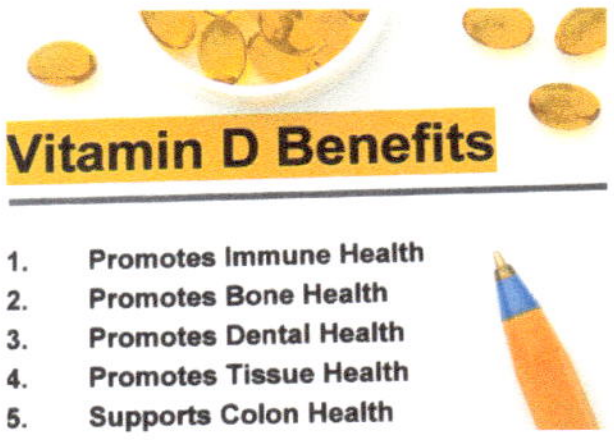

CALCIFEROL

Vit. D is critical to the absorption of calcium, phosphate & maximizing bone health. After the age of 50, bone breaks down faster that it forms a newborn. Bone loss often accelerates, especially during the time of menopause.

C

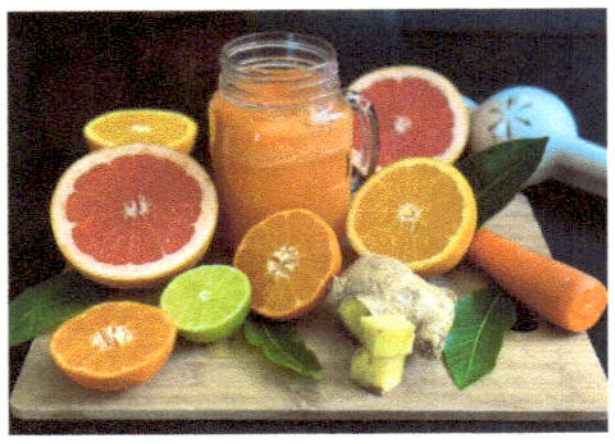

ASORBIC ACID

Vitamin C assists the body with forming blood vessels, muscle, cartilage & collagen in bones. It helps with the absorption of iron, functioning of the immune system, wound healing & more. Vitamin C also improves hormone levels.

B12

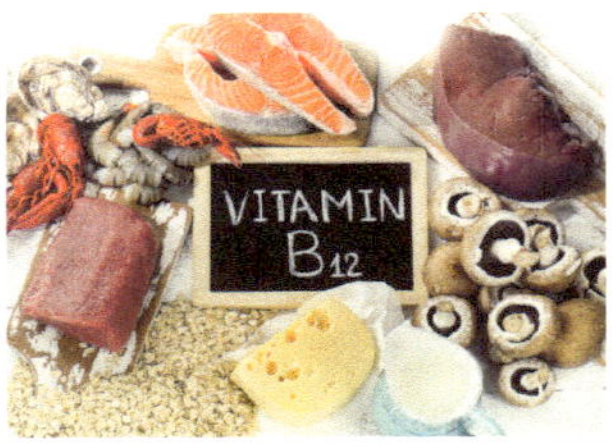

COBALAMIN; CYANOCOBALAMIN

B12 helps to create DNA, it is nourishment for the brain & nervous system. It improves energy levels, mood & vitality. It also supports bone health & boosts metabolism. Vitamin B12 & C should **not** be taken together. It is good to take B12 with magnesium to help with their absorption process.

A

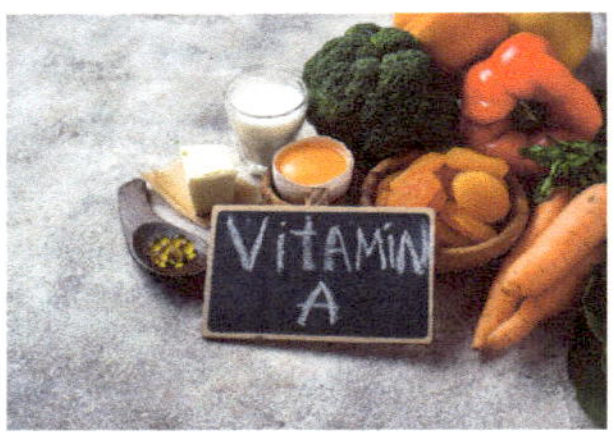

RETINOL

Excellent for vision. Helps to maintain skeletal & soft tissue, mucus membranes & skin. Also, it helps to maintain a healthy reproductive system. For pregnant and breastfeeding moms, vitamin A helps to build the immune system of the unborn child and the infant.

B2

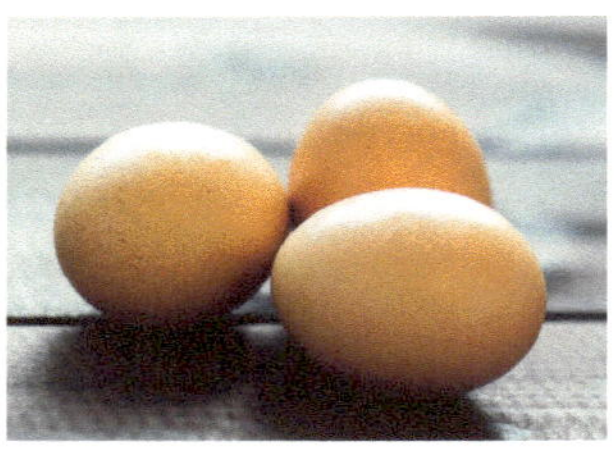

RIBOFLAVIN

B2 is an excellent vitamin. It reduces oxidative stress and inflammation of the nerves. It helps with the creation of red blood cells and releases energy from proteins. It converts food into fuel. We need B2 to properly use carbohydrates in our bodies.

B6

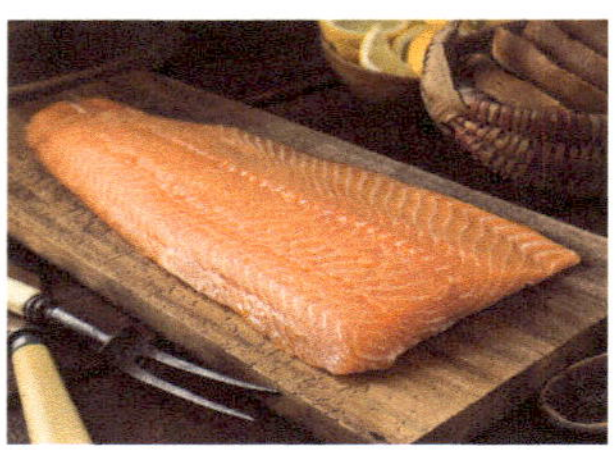

PYRIDOXINE

Vitamin B6 helps the body make antibodies. It promotes brain health & can help improve your mood. B6 also helps with metabolism, supports hair growth, slows down the greying of hair and can significantly reduce feelings of depression, anxiety and stress!

ESSENTIAL MINERALS FOR WOMEN

Ca

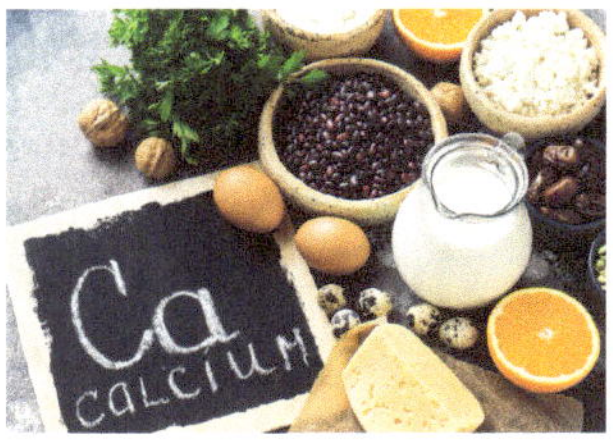

CALCIUM

Calcium & Vit. D work together to build strong bones. What people may not know is calcium fights kidney stones, helps to transport nutrients, balances PH levels in the body towards alkaline, and it plays a vital role in the electrical signaling of your heart. Women's bones are less dense than men, so we need more daily calcium intake.

Zn

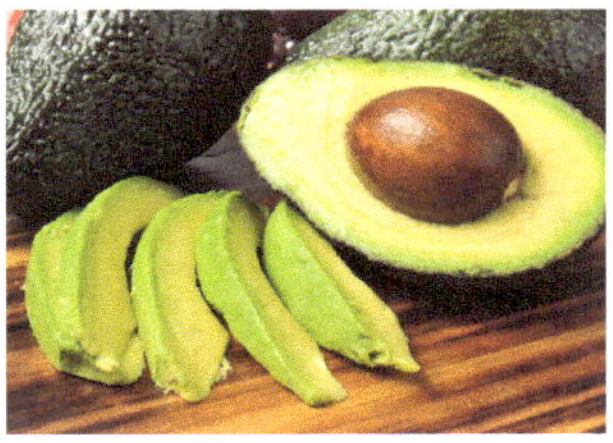

ZINC

Did you know zinc regulates a woman's cycle? After iron, zinc is the most abundant mineral in the body. It helps the immune system, wound healing, blood clotting, thyroid function & the sense of taste and smell. It also supports normal growth & development throughout life.

K

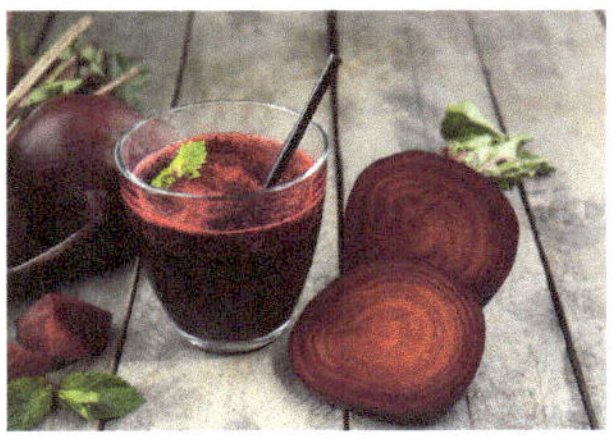

POTASSIUM

Potassium helps muscles to contract and supports normal blood pressure. It synthesizes protein & metabolizes carbohydrates. It also supports proper function of the nervous system. Sodium & potassium together maintain your fluid levels. Tip...Dried fruits are high in potassium.

Mg

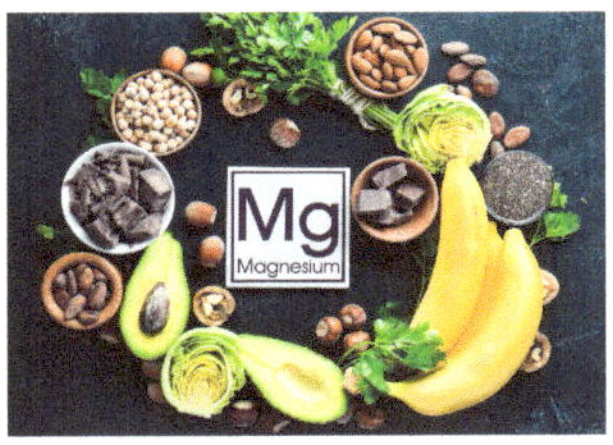

MAGNESIUM

Magnesium has a positive impact on hormonal health in the areas of sleep, PMS & mood. It helps to regulate levels of estrogen. Magnesium plays a critical role in nerve function, muscle support & energy production. It also activates the part of the nervous system that calms the body down.

Fe

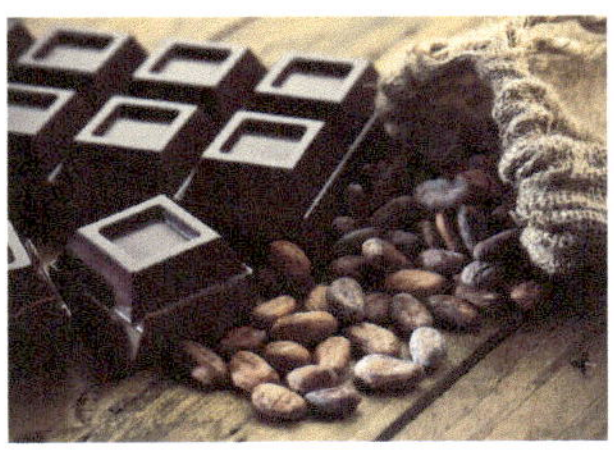

IRON

Iron carries oxygen through the blood. It helps to reduce tiredness, fatigue & normal energy metabolism. Iron also supports growth & development. Our bodies need iron to make certain hormones. Having ample amounts of iron in our bodies helps us to rest better at night.

Po

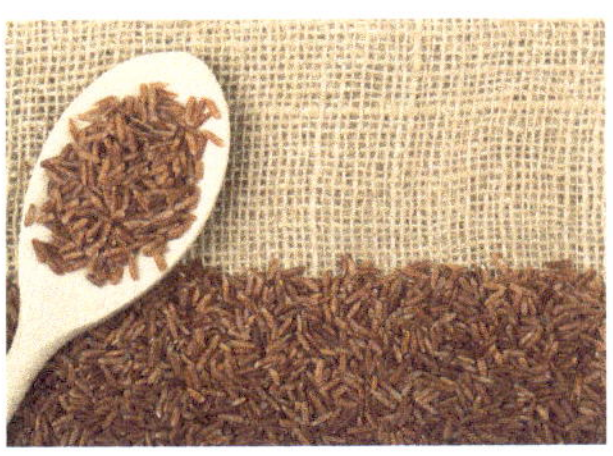

PHOSPHATE

Phosphate is needed for growth & repair of tissues & cells. It helps your nerves & muscles function. Calcium needs phosphorus to keep your bones & teeth strong. Phosphorus is a buffer that keeps blood pH balanced. It also helps us to turn fat, carbs & protein into energy. Phosphorus is a part of what makes our DNA.

CHECK IN POINT

WHAT CAN YOU IMMEDIATELY INCORPORATE INTO YOUR LIFE FROM THIS READING?

STEPS OF ACTION

WHAT MENTAL HEALTH CHANGES ARE YOU INSPIRED TO DO?

STEPS TO ACTION

Mindfulness

Creating A Better You In This Moment

The Power Is In Your Hands

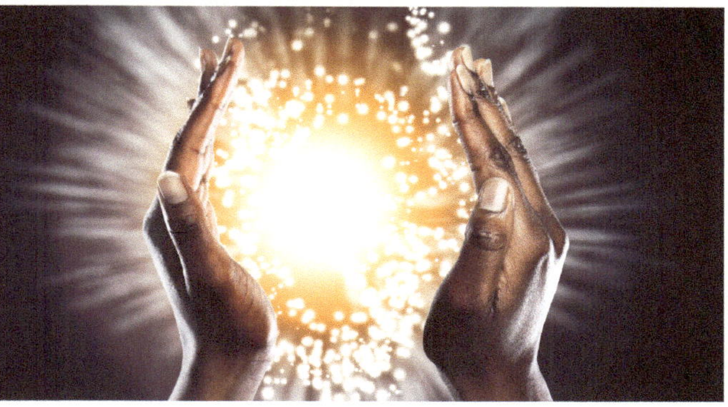

YOUR STRENTHS	YOUR TEMP WEAKNESSES

Self Care Checklist

WHAT NEEDS TO BE ON YOUR LIST?

- TRY SOMETHING NEW
- GO ON A NATURE WALK
- MEDITATE
- MAKE A VISION BOARD
- CONNECT WITH FRIENDS
- WATCH YOUR FAV MOVIE
- HAVE A LONG NAP
- GIVE YOURSELF CREDIT
- PRACTICE DEEP BREATHING
- DRINK SOME HERBAL TEA
- PLAN A FUN DAY OUT
- CALL A FAMILY MEMBER
- WRITE IN A JOURNAL
- COOK YOUR FAV FOOD
- LIGHT A CANDLE
- CREATE A QUIET/TRUSTED SPACE
- COMPLIMENT YOURSELF
- DANCE TO MUSIC
- EAT NOURISHING FOOD
- GO TO A WORKOUT CLASS
- TAKE A BREAK
- BUY SOMETHING YOU DESERVE
- READ A BOOK
- **SAY YES TO YOURSELF**
- CREATE AFFIRMATIONS
- DECLUTTER YOUR MIND

NOTE TO SELF

CHALLENGE

BALANCE IS SO IMPORTANT, EVERY MONTH TRY AND SCHEDULE THESE SELF-CARE CHALLENGES

- Create a daily schedule that includes self-care activities.
- List your guilt factors and eliminate them.
- Give up one bad habit for 30 days.
- Eat a healthy meal without distractions.
- Attend a musical or a play.
- Go on a mindful nature walk.
- Begin removing your fears one at a time.
- Get a full check up from your doctors office.
- Rest properly for seven to eight hours.
- Release your daily stress before bed.

Date :

Day :

Note :

Daily Planner

TODAY'S PLAN

TO DO LIST

REMINDER

APPOINTMENT

TODAY IN ONE WORD

New Mood

New Me

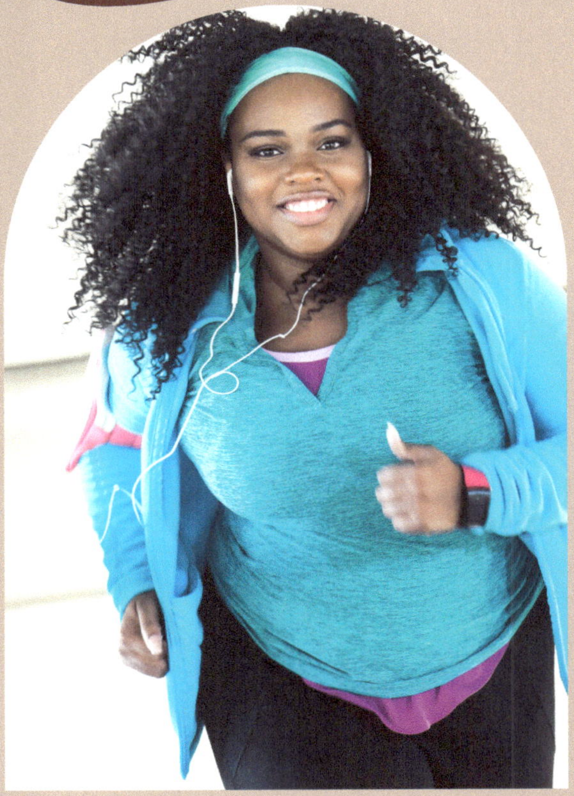

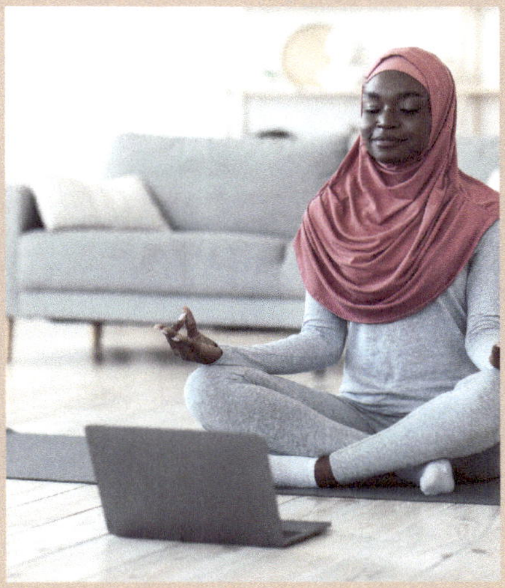

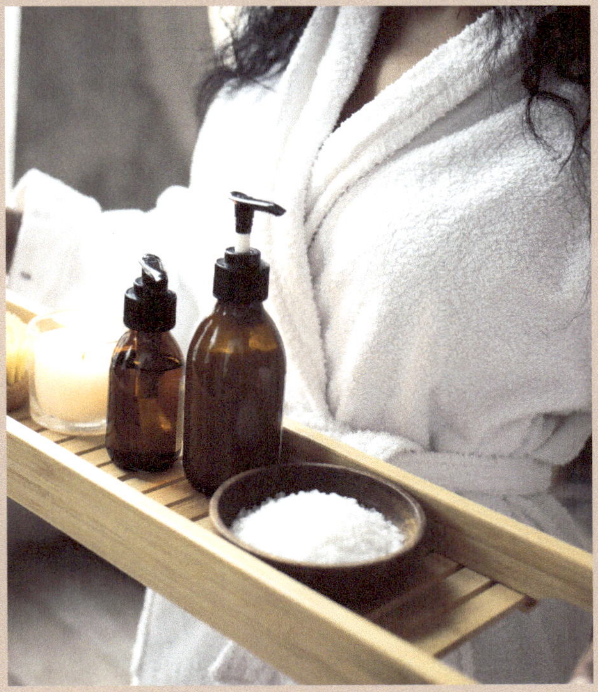

New Reality

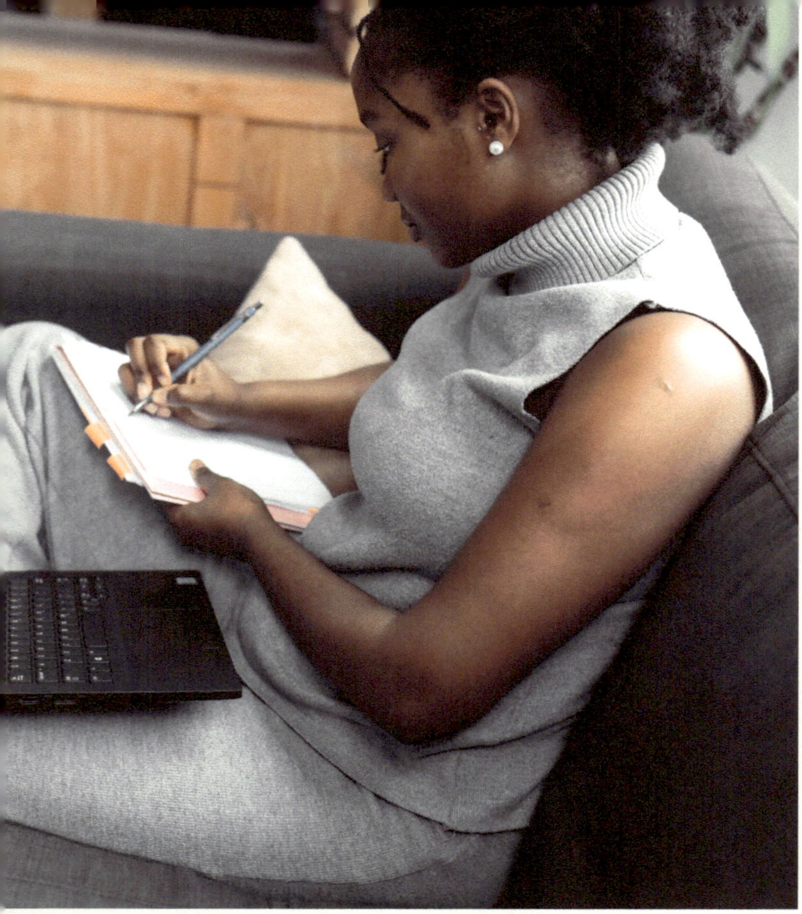

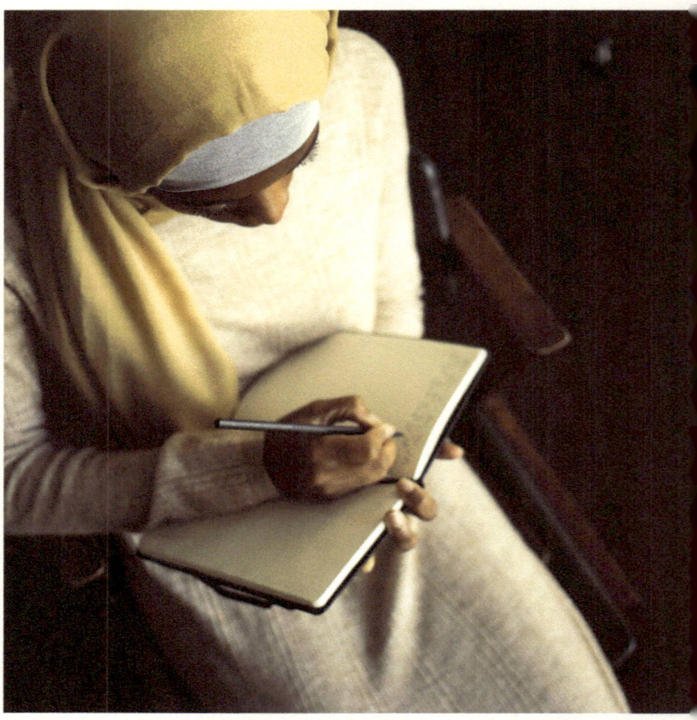

Gratitude Journal

PRACTICE GRATITUDE BEFORE YOU GO TO BED AT NIGHT

Taking a moment to recognize the good things in life allows us to take a mental note of how blessed we really are. It allows our emotional tone to shift in profound ways.

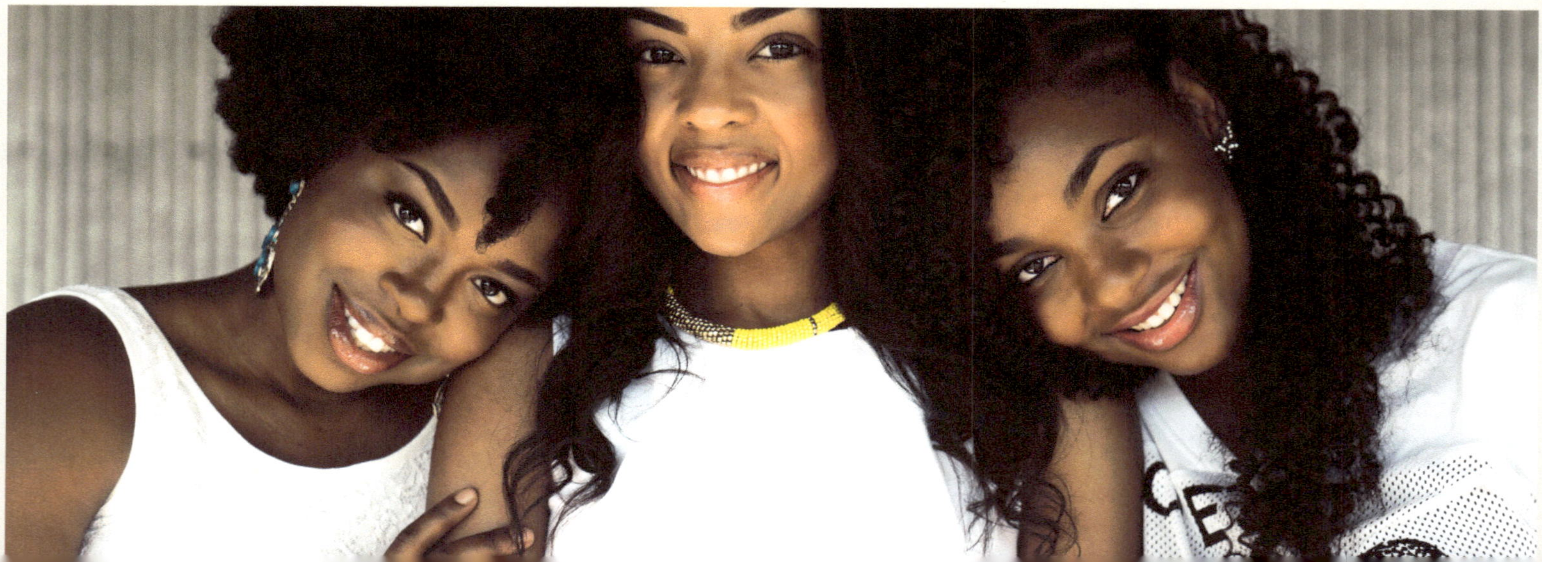

DATE

Mood

DAILY JOURNAL

YOUR THOUGHTS

GOALS

TO DO

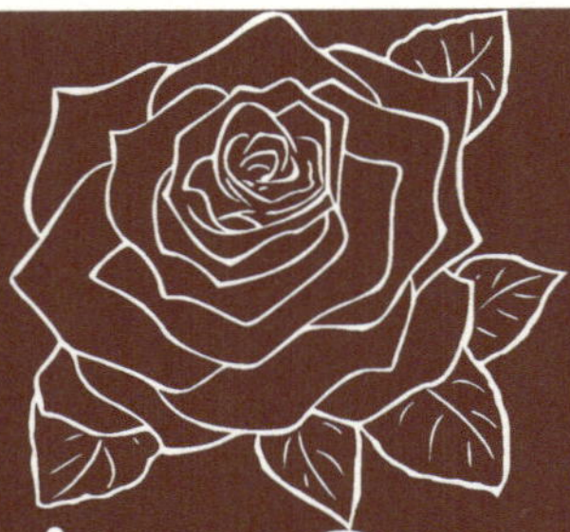

Evening Gratitude

3 things I'm grateful for today are...

The best part of today was...

What can I learn from today's experiences?

Tomorrow I'm looking forward to...

Do more of what you love. You deserve it!

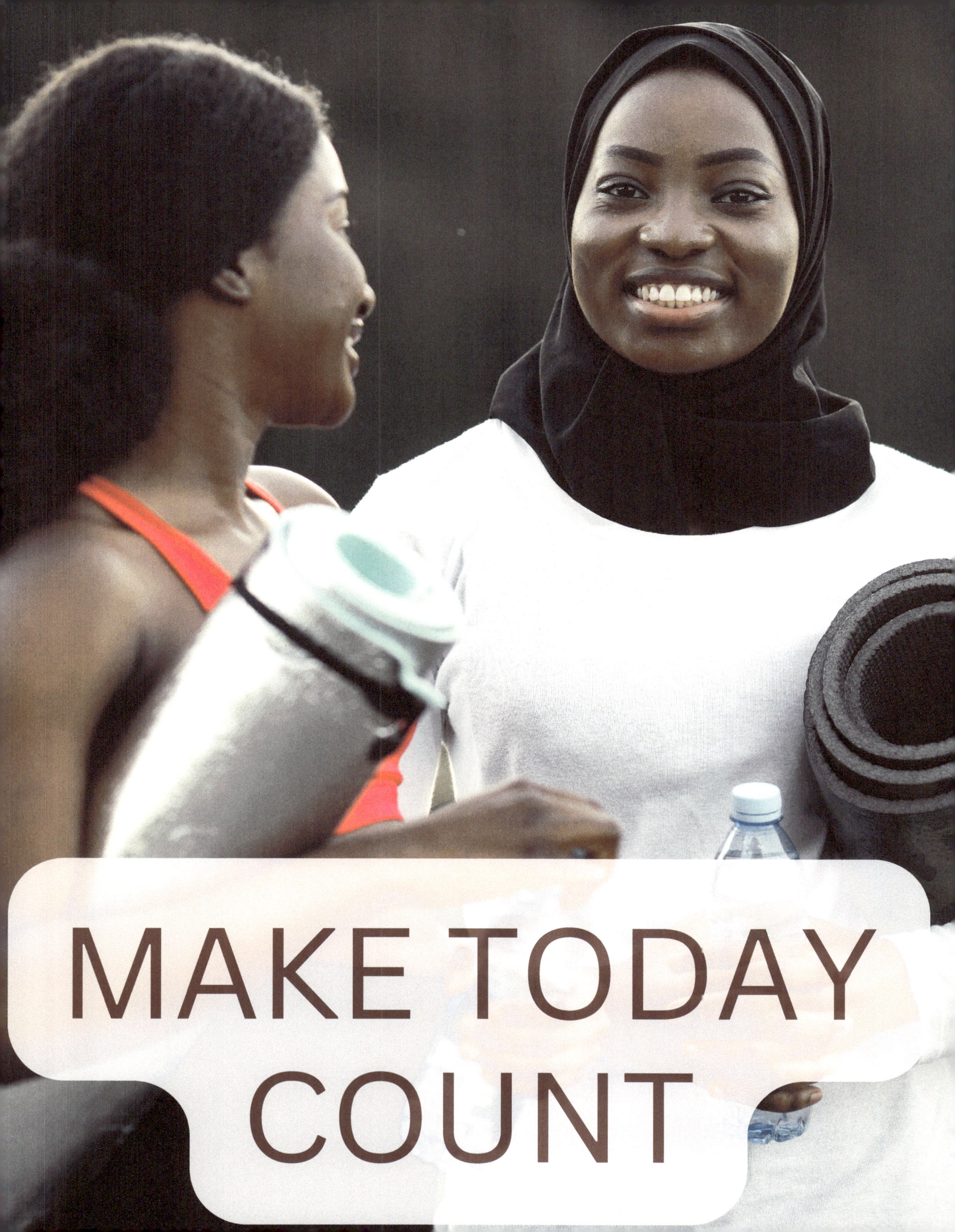
MAKE TODAY
COUNT

Bibliography

Center for Disease Control and Prevention, "Common Reproductive Health Concerns for Women," April, 27, 2918, CDC.com

Center for Disease Control and Prevention, "Cholesterol," March 20, 2023, CDC.com

Levine GN, Lange RA, Bairey-Merz CN, et al. Meditation and cardiovascular risk reduction: a scientific statement from the American Heart Association. Journal of the American Heart Association. 2017;6(10):e002218.

Johnson, Traci C, WebMed, "Vitamins Women Need", April 23, 2023, webmd.com

Salamon, Maureen, "Surprising Foods That Boosts Bone Health," Harvard Health Publishing, January 1, 2023, health.harvard.edu

Lakhiani, Vishen, *The Code of the Extraordinary Mind,* United States, Rodale Books, 2016

Mayer MD, Emeran, *The Mind-Gut Connection*, New York, NY, Harper Collins Publishers, 2016

Li, William W., *Eat To Beat Disease*, New York, NY, Grand Central Publishing, 2019

Mosconi PhD, Lisa, *Brain Food*, New York, NY, Penguin Random House LLC, 2018

Swift, Katja, *Herbal Medicine for Beginners,* Emeryville, Ca, Althea Press, 2018

MORE PUBLICATIONS

01 WHY I AM ENOUGH

Your daily inspiration! This book is power packed with comfort and healing. You can carry it with you wherever you go!

ORDER YOUR COPY
WWW.HTLC19.ORG

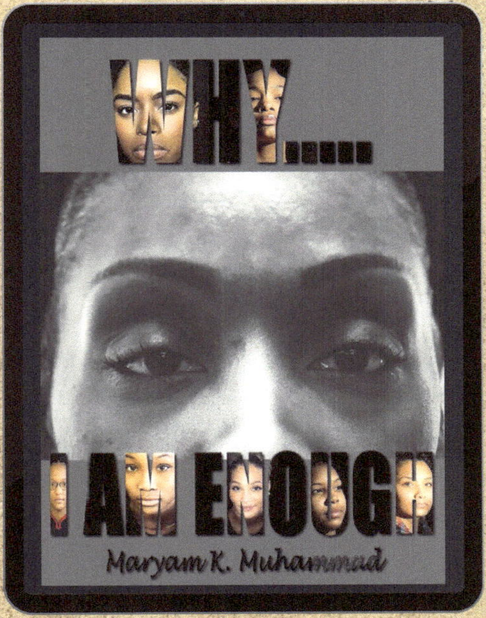

02 THE POWER TO BREAK GENERATIONAL PAIN

This book is the process to unplug ourselves from the pain of our past. "Your Healing Workbook" is the practical application of this book.

ORDER YOUR COPY
WWW.HTLC19.ORG

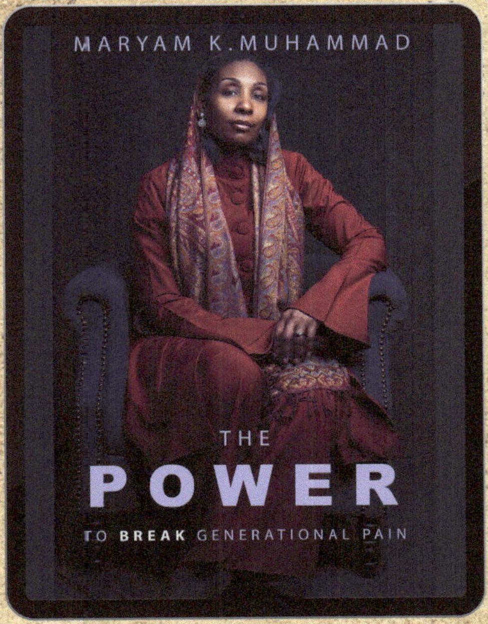

MORE PUBLICATIONS

03 YOUR HEALING WORKBOOK

This book is designed to equip you with the tools and tips needed to release you from your past pain so that you may live the life you deserve to live!

ORDER YOUR COPY
WWW.HTLC19.ORG

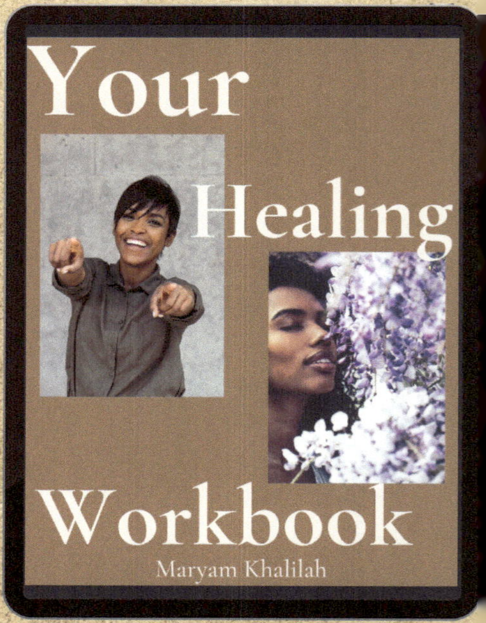

THANK YOU!

I thank God for blessing me with the mind and guidance to create this workbook for you. I am not the healer, God is! I thank you for being courageous enough to take the steps to heal your life. Always keep God in mind. Remember, when your inner self awakens and removes insecurities and you strengthen your self-love, you are on your way to living a healthier lifestyle.

You were born on purpose with a purpose. God has a plan for you. Walk with Him. His essence is in you. Pull on it and use it. Only settle on God's energy from this day forward!

Claim your victory. You're already winning!

Maryam Khalilah

xoxo

STAY IN TOUCH

INSTAGRAM @HTLC19

TWITTER @HTLC19

WWW.HTLC19.ORG

FACEBOOK @HTLC19

www.ingramcontent.com/pod-product-compliance
Ingram Content Group UK Ltd.
Pitfield, Milton Keynes, MK11 3LW, UK
UKHW060015051026
15591UKWH00002B/223